The Secrets to Long Life

How to Live Life Beyond 100 Years

Charles Tita

Published by New Generation Publishing in 2021

First Edition

Paperback ISBN: 978-1-80031-425-2
Hardback ISBN: 978-1-80031-424-5

www.newgeneration-publishing.com

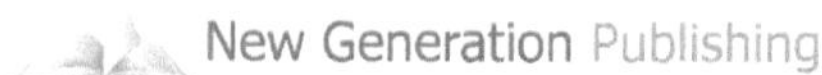

Foreword

Knowledge is power! If you've never believed in the eternal wisdom of that popular aphorism, trust me, you will, after reading this book. The value of any intellectual pursuit lies in its ability to transform our lives, by stimulating our minds, making us to think differently and hopefully enriching our collective experience.

When I first got invited to write the foreword to a self-help book on health or alternative medicine, titled, *"How to Live Pain-free to 100 Years and Beyond",* nothing could have been more revolting to me. My first instinct was an outright refusal; for I've been a lifelong, dedicated, and cold-hearted critic of the genre. It felt like I'd just been asked to relive my worst nightmares.

Let me explain. Perish the thought, but imagine if someone murdered your parents, and at their funeral, you were asked to say nice things about their killer. That is exactly how I've always felt about certain self-help books. I was personally tormented by the suggestion of writing the foreword for the type of literature about which I have always held a healthy aversion and regarded with great contempt and disdain. My perception of motivational literature on health used to border on scepticism, for the simple reason that I always considered them as pseudo-scientific quackery. The overriding perception was that many of such handbooks were written by hawk-eyed opportunists and quacks, with a dewy-eyed gaze for financial gain, and very little consideration for how their books would be beneficial to their readers.

In recent years, not a single self-help book written has given me any cause to clamber to my feet and give it a rousing cheer. Hence, even as I grudgingly accepted the challenge to just, "*read the book, and say whatever you disliked about it,"* I knew that I was only going to read it with a very critical eye to correct all the grammar, pick holes in it, and dismiss it as another mediocre literature concocted by a starving author—like myself. Even the title of the book seemed overly ambitious and exaggerated to me, with an air of audacious arrogance. I was even less impressed with the tag-line—The Vital Life Force.

How can anyone claim to have the panacea for near immortality—to have the secrets of living beyond 100 years, was my question.

How wrong was I.

As it has been widely stated, the taste of the pudding lies in the eating. And until I actually began to read the book, I didn't realise what valuable lessons I had missed and what I was actually gaining from it. The first teaching moment while reading was that, contrary to popular beliefs, first impressions are not always right. I was humbled by the immensity of the knowledge I found therein, after just a few pages of reading and from that moment on, I was converted from a strident critic to an instant admirer.

Occasionally, a book comes along that simply responds to the needs of our time. It answers those perennial questions that have always eluded us, giving us the hope that there is a possibility that at any age, we can change the course of our existence and improve our circumstances. And as I started reading; right from the very start of the book, I just knew that I had something special in my hands. It was like finding a gem— a gem hiding in the mud, picking it up, and running it under tap water and discovering a glistening rare diamond.

The second lesson I learned while reading the book was that I didn't even have to buy it afterwards. I started practising what I had discovered from the vast array of information, as they unfolded before my eyes—which is a testament to how easily practical the guidelines are. I tried the simple techniques provided and instantly discovered their usefulness. I felt lucky that I had been chosen to have a foretaste of valuable knowledge which others were going to pay a princely sum to have. My eyes were eventually opened to the fact that even if I felt good about my overall health, there are things I could still do to improve myself, for we are all susceptible to the aging process. Therefore, regardless of the general state of anyone's health, as long as you live, there are things you need to monitor and improve about yourself in order to avoid the inevitable pains of growing old.

I also discovered to my great delight that the audacity of the title was not a far-fetched exaggeration, as it first appeared to me. It seemed as if the writer had discovered a treasure trove of information which once belonged to an exclusive club of health scientists, and was sharing it with ordinary mortals. Those who are familiar with Greek mythology may remember the cult figure called Prometheus. Prometheus was known for his intelligence and generosity. As a cultural icon, he was celebrated as the champion of mankind for his selfless act of heroism, for he stole fire from the Greek gods and gave it to mankind, which helped humans to build a strong civilisation. This book was almost akin to that sort of mythology—a daring benevolent gesture by a doughty researcher who discovered the secrets of good health, which will help us avoid the costly trips to the doctors, or the toxic requirements of swallowing multiple pills to keep us alive. You can add life to your years if you just try.

The author argues most eloquently, to express an advocacy for a disease-free existence, unencumbered by pain and suffering for a long time—beyond 100 years. That life is beautiful is without doubt. But that it is possible to be enjoyed if we followed the secrets that he has divulged in this book, means we have been handed the power to improve our lives. By practising the simple steps as advised, we may have bought for ourselves another 25 years of life or even more. There is no panacea for immortality but it is possible to live a quality existence that doesn't require costly trips to the doctors or the need to break our bank accounts just to keep us alive. The best part of this is, there is no time limit given for anyone to start improving their health and there is a choice available for everyone to pace themselves according to their own circumstances.

Inside this book, you'll learn things about yourself you took for granted, and also about the diseases that frequently afflict mankind. He provides little practical steps to help you to improve the quality of your organs and hormonal balances that keep you functioning like a well-oiled machine. You will discover the cyclical patterns of our lives that affect us. Like the fact that your mood directly affects your weight gain, as much as your hormonal balances. That the presence of hormones like cortisol cause the stress that affects your moods in the first place. He also provides the answers to how you could avoid the negative imbalances that are bad for your health, while prescribing the simple things you can do to avoid the number one killer; cardiovascular diseases like heart attacks and strokes.

You will also learn how good health is directly connected to your sex drive.

When I was done reading the book, my first impression was: I wish someone had written this book when I was in my twenties or younger. I would've been in the best possible shape and form of my life today.

Something beautiful about the book is the simplicity of its language. It is written in a straightforward and simple English, which helps every reader to understand what is required to achieve their mission, while avoiding the clump of medical lingo that often confuses the reader.

At a time when our world is facing an existential health crisis; with the worst plague that has hit mankind, with no cure in sight, the best thing anyone could hope for is to prepare their bodies to be fit enough to withstand any diseases, without suffering too much. A stitch in time saves nine. There's no better preparation anyone could do than to invest in their health.

If you were a self-help sceptic like I was, I urge you to get yourself a copy of the book and discover for yourself. The secrets of how to live a pain-free existence beyond 100 years is no longer a secret. It is contained in this book.

Introduction

The world is full of a vast array of diseases and illnesses which have left humanity crippled with unnecessary pain and suffering. Today, we have pathologies and maladies which seem incurable. Luckily, in our interconnected world replete with information, invaluable knowledge about cures and pain-relief, which were once held in the mystified realms of a selected few, can now be revealed and shared to all those who really need it.

Do you know that you can live a healthy, happy, successful, long and productive life, well beyond the average life expectancy? The secrets all lie within a robust immune system, which helps our bodies to fight diseases. We can identify, isolate and prevent pathologies even before they manifest themselves in our bodies, if only we knew how to build our immune systems to be strong enough to fight these crushing illnesses. We know that very dangerous viruses and bacteria can cause us to get sick and there are diseases that have the potential to threaten the very survival of humanity itself. Luckily, we have the ability to prevent that kind of catastrophic scenario.

In this study, we will reveal to you the secrets of the natural laws that will enable you to live disease-free for 100 years and more, with very little or no medication at all. It can be done if only you followed our instructions judiciously.

Our teachings are designed to serve as pillars of support for you to follow, in your quest to live a wholesome, healthy and happy life for a very long time, as long as you follow our simple instructions. You will be able to transform yourself into an enviable state of being, bursting full with life, blossoming with *vigour and vitality*. In order to attain this state of wellbeing, you would have followed our guidelines, with an understanding to appreciate the legacy of ancient wisdom handed over to us by the great masters of an epoch that is past.

The root of all life forms is the **Absolute**. The Absolute, which we generally call "God" cannot be conceived. From this ineffable Absolute, there emanates an eternal energy called the Vital Life Force, which constitutes the great arcana, or the mysteries of our collective humanity. In this Vital Life Force lies the hidden secrets that can enable everyone to live a healthy, happy long life, free of sickness and pain.

A staggering number of books have been written about health, but very little is still known about the most important energy that sustains the human life itself. This time, we are letting the hidden secrets be known to everyone. The Vital Life Force is a Living Power; the power of life. Every living thing, big or small is infused with this vital energy. If you want to know more about this energy, and how to use it to prevent all pathological conditions from which man may suffer, then read on.

CHAPTER ONE

Welcome to the heritage of natural health. In this first chapter we are going to present to you the causes of all pathologies with which mankind is heavily afflicted. We are also going to show you how to prevent all of them. It is with great joy that we welcome you and introduce you to this illustrious and fragrant path of an ancient wisdom.

Count yourself lucky to be among those who can assess this knowledge. The objective of this teaching is to give to you the means to live a disease-free existence to a ripe old age, during which you will also be very healthy and very happy.

WHAT IS LIFE?

What sustains human life is a combination of two mutually symbiotic energies. As we mentioned in the introduction, they are the Positive Vital Life Force and the Negative Vital Life Force.

The Positive Vital Life Force emanates from above, and it is found in the **air we breathe**, and it is an energy which is especially concentrated in our cell's nucleus. Meanwhile, the Negative Vital Life Force is brought into the body by the **food and the drinks we ingest,** and it is held in the small intestine, from which the bloodstream becomes the carrier of its corresponding energy. The Negative Vital Life Force is mostly concentrated in the exterior membrane of each cell.

We read from the good book that in the beginning, God took the dust; which is the Negative Vital Life Force, and breathed into man the Breath of Life. And so, man became a living being. Therefore, life as it is found on earth is the manifestation of that energy that we have already mentioned above, which the Ancient Masters called the Vital Life Force. This energy comes into the body at the moment of our birth, when the newborn child takes in its first breath. Death occurs at the time of the last breath, for it is then that this Vital Life Force departs from the human body.

CAUSES OF ILLNESSES

For a natural, healthy life to exist there must be a balanced combination of the two Positive and Negative Vital Life Energies in the human body. The fact that we have presented this great principle in a rather simple manner does not negate its essence or downplay its importance to human existence. The cause of all illnesses is when there is an imbalance of these two energies in the human body. Though there are harmful bacteria and viruses, it is difficult for them to penetrate a body which has a robust balance of both the Positive and the Negative Vital Life Forces.

Even when diseases manage to penetrate the human body, it will be able to fight them off, with very little or no medical assistance. We know of individuals who have come in contact with patients who are afflicted with deadly viruses but were not contaminated themselves because they had a very robust immune system.

Sickness and pain only come in when there is an imbalance of these two energies in the human body. The lack of this equilibrium affects all other parts of the body. Pain and suffering are the results of all illnesses. Those who are aware of this vital principle of harmony and balance will never stray from this equilibrium. It helps them to revitalise and recreate themselves. They will maintain it and will find eternal happiness. They will remain in harmony with life, and be able to create and recreate themselves constantly and keep illnesses at bay.

But those whose bodies lack this equilibrium, who often violate the laws and the balance of life as a result of ignorance, will endure pain and suffering on themselves.

Medicine is founded in nature. Nature herself is medicine, and only in her shall mankind seek its cures. Nature is the physician's teacher, for she is older than the physician. The most effective therapies or the cures for diseases are those which are most compatible with the laws of nature.

There are two kinds of health: the natural and the artificial. Scientific medicine has gifted mankind with artificial health and protection against most infectious diseases. It is a marvellous gift. But humans cannot contend with a life devoid of malady that is sustained by special diets, chemicals, endocrine products, vitamins, periodic medical examinations, expensive trips to the hospitals, doctors, and nurses. Humans want to stay naturally healthy, which comes from the body's inherent ability to resist infectious, degenerative diseases and viruses.

The purpose of this book is therefore to help to furnish you with the know-how to prevent all infections. You will learn how to keep degenerative diseases and opportunistic viruses and infections away, while living a natural and healthy life. it is well known that artificial health does not suffice for human happiness and medical care is often very costly and can sometime prove to be ineffective.

Even though people often appear in great health, the wear and tear of the human body that occur over time means that the body is always in constant need of small or large repairs. Sometimes this repair mechanism may not be sufficient to put the human body back into it previous form, in which it was strong and fully healthy. Everyone would agree that happiness cannot be enjoyed when one is experiencing pain in one's body.

Another lesson you will learn from this book is that it will enable you to better comprehend the origins of all pathologies from which mankind suffer. You will be given a full understanding of the simple natural tools that you will need to maintain good health and remain in a state of harmony with your body that is as perfect as is naturally possible.

Before we tell you all you need to know about the Positive and Negative Vital Life Forces and how to use them, we want to remind you once more that all diseases that have been diagnosed and catalogued are caused by a single fundamental cause; lack of the body's harmony. If there is a lack of balance between the Positive and Negative Vital Life Forces in the human body, it will create a fundamental disharmony in the entire mechanism and decrease the vibrant frequency of our existence.

Do not ever forget this great principle. When these two energies are not balanced in the body, we tend to be weak and open to illnesses. Our entire vibratory energy at this point becomes low, making us vulnerable to such pathogenic agents in the environment as germs, viruses, fungi and bacteria.

After much research, we are convinced that the day will come when the veracity of this principle will be widely recognised as the most effective form of preventing illnesses. This type of natural remedy will one day offer mankind its greatest hope, as far as healing is concerned, and the time to sow the seeds of its efficacy is right now.

THE POSITIVE VITAL LIFE FORCE

The Positive Vital Life Force, as earlier stated, is found in the air we breathe. The Vital Life Force in the air; which we here designate as the Positive Energy, is the essence of all motions, forces and energies, whether manifested in gravitation, electricity, the revolution of the planets or all forms of life—from the lowest to the highest.

In order to be free of all infections or from all opportunistic pathologies which we may sometimes be unable to avoid, we need to know how to use the Positive Vital Life Force to its greatest advantage to infection and transmission. This great principle which we designate as a Positive Energy is in the air, but it is not the air, nor one of its chemical constituents. Animal and plant life breathe it in with the air, and yet, if the air did not contain it, they would die, even though they might be filled with air. It is taken up by the system along with the oxygen, and yet it is not the oxygen.

The Hebrew writer of the Book of Genesis knew the difference between the atmospheric air, and the Mysterious Potential Principle contained within it. He speaks of *neshemet rush chayin;* which when translated means, "The breath of the spirit of life." It is the same as the Vital Life Force. Ancient philosophers have known that breathing is a significant function and that its usefulness is far from being limited to the gaseous exchanges produced in the lungs.

The breathing exercise was an art form that was practised in Ancient Egypt. At about the same time, it became an integral part of the religious practices to which Brahmins in India devoted themselves on a daily basis; practices which are the sources of the current forms of Yoga today.

As there are different types of diets, so are there different types of breathing. In fact, there are three types of breathing. Deep breathing, negative breathing and shallow breathing.

- Deep breathing enables us to take in enough Positive Vital Life Force into the body.
- Negative breathing helps to get rid of the toxins in the body. It helps to expel the portion of the carbon dioxide produced in the lungs.
- Shallow breathing is neutral or normal breathing.
- Deep breathing plays a critical role in the energy balance, which we must maintain through our entire body.

Hundreds of books have been written on diet, the source of the Negative Vital Life Force, but very few have been written on deep breathing, the source of the Positive Vital Life Force. Deep breathing is equally as important as a good diet.

DEEP BREATHING EXERCISE

Breathing is one of the most important functions of the human body because the lungs are truly the seat of vital breath, and consequently, of the essential aspect of the Life Energy which animates them. To obtain and maintain a good amount of the Positive Vital Life Force needed in the body, we need deep breathing. At this point, it would be very useful to give you an exercise on how to take in enough Positive Vital Life Force using deep breathing.

Experiment No.1

We suggest that you perform this exercise at anytime you feel the need for physical or mental regeneration. You're advised to perform it in the morning when you wake up, in order to diminish the body's toxicity, as it puts you in a good mood at the very start of the day. This exercise will not only strengthen all the parts of your body, but your brain will receive an increase in its energy levels. Your latent faculties will be developed and psychic powers will be optimised.

This exercise is particularly important for people like students, to help them regenerate and boost their mental faculty. People who master the science of storing enough Positive Vital Life Energy in the body, consciously or unconsciously, always radiate vitality and strength. This strength cannot be missed by those with whom they come in contact. Such a person may project this strength to others and give them an increase in their own vitality and health. The exercise, called "*Magnetic Healing*" is performed in this way, although many practitioners are not aware of the source of their power.

Do the following:

1. Sit down on a chair, with your back as straight as possible, your feet flat on the floor, slightly apart from each other, and place your palms on your knees.

2. Now breathe out all the air in your lungs through the nose, and force the last remaining air in your lungs out through the mouth.
3. Immediately after doing this, inhale slowly and deeply for about 15 seconds or above; as if you want to take in all the air in the atmosphere.
4. Expand your chest and stomach with air.
5. Now hold the air in your lungs for about 25 seconds, or for as long as you can without discomfort. Then slowly exhale fully through the nose, emptying all the air in your lungs and finally forcing out the last remaining air in your lungs out through your mouth.
6. Repeat this deep breathing exercise for about five to ten minutes, or after repeating this type of breathing for about eight to nine time, stand up and resume your normal daily activities.

This deep breathing exercise is equal to more than thirty minutes of vigorous workout, as it has lots of other benefits.

Deep breathing is the oxygenation process to all of the cells in the body. It is generally used as a natural pain killer. Deep breathing is the only means by which we can obtain enough Positive Vital Life Force, but very few people are aware of this very important function to their health. Deep breathing improves blood flow, increases energy level, improves your posture, reduces inflammation, detoxifies your body, stimulates the lymphatic system, improves your digestion, relaxes mind and body, increases your libido, calms your nervous system and releases muscle tension. It improves the cardiovascular system and generally keeps our bodies youthful.

Deep breathing also slows the aging process by increasing the secretion of anti-aging hormones, with the help of the aforementioned Positive Vital Life Force. It has been discovered that people who practice deep breathing have longer telomeres; which are the protective caps found at the end of chromosomes in the human body. Short telomeres have been linked to premature cellular aging. Deep breathing generally helps to strengthen the immune system.

If you fail to breathe in deeply and properly, you won't be able to get rid of the toxins in your system and this is exactly what leads to illnesses. Lack of deep breathing is a problem that too many people are facing. Many people do not realise that their breathing is shallow. When your breathing is shallow, you can't get the right amount of oxygen or the Positive Vital Life Force that your body requires to keep you healthy. Your body becomes weak, tensed, stressed and constricted. This is a function that is neglected by most people.

When we fail to breathe properly, our inhalation is generally too weak; and subsequently, we reduce the quantity of the Positive Vital Life Force needed by our bodies. Our exhalation is also often insufficient to expel the portion of the carbon dioxide produced by the body. This un-expelled carbon dioxide often accumulates in the inferior lobes of our lungs, engendering any number of negative consequences to our system.

Of all the essential functions which ensure the life of a living physical organism, breathing is the most constant. Humans can live for many days without food. They may also go for a day or two without sleep, but no human can stay for more than five minutes without breathing. Immediately one stops breathing the Positive Vital Life Force disconnects and the human ceases to exist.

No life is can be sustained without the Positive Vital Life Force. Of all the functions of the human organism, the respiratory system is the one which must be guarded the most and the one which must be given priority. We must understand that bad ventilation of the respiratory apparatus entails self-intoxication and that is in a nutshell the cause of many health problems. We must therefore learn how to breathe deeply, so as to increase the resistance of the human organs and in order to build our strength for all times.

NEGATIVE BREATHING

Experiment No.2

1. Stand straight up with your legs touching each other and your hands by your sides.
2. While standing in that position, breath out all the air in your lungs slowly and deeply.
3. After taking out all the air in your lungs, hold your breath without breathing in for about 20 seconds for as long as you can without any discomfort.
4. Then breathe in slowly and deeply; and again breathe out all the air in your lungs and hold your breath without breathing in.
5. After holding your breath for as long as you can without discomfort, breathe in slowly.
6. Repeat this process for about five times. Then continue with your normal breathing.

It is advisable to perform this negative breathing before the deep breathing exercise. Negative breathing helps to expel toxins in the body and detoxify the cells. It is necessary to do this exercise whenever you feel a rise in your body temperature.

Now that you are aware of the importance of deep breathing, we advise that you take up any form of physical exercise or sports of your choice. Regular deep breathing exercises lower the risk of heart disease, stroke and diabetes. A healthier heart means a reduced risk of cardiovascular diseases. It improves sleep and can battle any feelings of anxiety and depression, sharpen and improve your self-esteem. When we add all these benefits above what do we get? A longer, healthier and more enjoyable life.

THE NEGATIVE VITAL LIFE FORCE

As we've already discussed, life on earth as we know it is a manifestation of a universal energy called Vital Life Force.

Wikipedia defines this Vital Life Force as, "*Vitalism, the ability to live or exist. An active principle forming part of any living thing*".

As previously mentioned, the phrase Vital Life Force has two phases; the Positive and the Negative.

Life on earth cannot exist without these two polarities. The Positive Vital Life Force as stated, is found in the air we breathe, while the Negative Vital Life Force is found in plants, water and all living organisms on planet earth. The Negative phase of the Vital Life Force is linked to the food and drinks we absorb into our bodies.

Ultimately, if we do not eat or drink sufficiently, our bodies will be in a state of imbalance. As it is also true with breathing, many people observe very bad diet habits, because their meals are not nutritionally balanced. There is increasing evidence that a particular type of diet is the best for the human body and brain function. A diet that is rich in vegetables, whole grains, and healthy fats has been recognised as the healthiest for the human brain and body. This diet is known by different names; including "plant based" and "Mediterranean". But at its core, it is focused on vegetables, protein, and healthy fats.

The US news and World Report recently ranked the Mediterranean diet as the best to diet to follow in the years ahead. In a world dominated by celebrity fad diets, many people don't believe that there's a single best-diet for human health. But a growing body of research-based evidence suggests that a meal plan that is loaded with vegetables, proteins, and healthy fats has key benefits for losing weight, keeping the mind sharp while protecting the human heart and brain from age-related diseases.

Since the beginning of time, herbs have been an integral part of all life forms, human, animal and vegetation. Not only did herbs provide most of the earliest food sources for our ancestors, but also the medicines for their illnesses. They can also affect our moods and how we feel. Herbs gave birth to medicines which in turn paved the way for the modern pharmaceutical industry. Herbs, of course, are an integral part in modern medicine, both in Eastern practices and throughout the entire world.

There are many herbs today which are being taken for granted by some people, which were once known to be used effectively by ancient physicians and apothecaries in the East, many centuries ago, long before they became a part of Western pharmacopeia. The magical power of herbs held a divine essence to early humans. We find the reference, "*...and God said..., behold, I have given you every herb that is upon the face of the earth,*" Genesis (1:29).

As already mentioned in previous sections of this writeup, the Negative Vital Life Force is brought to the body by the food and drink we ingest. It is at the level of the small intestine that the bloodstream becomes the carrier of this corresponding energy. The Negative Vital Life Force is mostly concentrated in the exterior membrane of each cell.

In 2019 the US News and World Report released a list of best and worst diets; an annual ranking compiled by health and nutrition experts. In 2018, the Dash Diet and Mediterranean diet were tied for the first place on the list of best diets. But in 2019, the Mediterranean diet stood alone at the top of the list, thanks to research that linked it to longer and healthier lives.

What is the Dash Diet? The Dash Diet stands for Dietary Approaches to Stop Hypertension. It is promoted by the National Heart, Lungs, and Blood Institute to stop or prevent hypertension, otherwise known as high blood pressure. It **encourages** eating the foods you've have always been told to eat regularly; fruits, veggies, whole grains, lean protein and low-fat dairy, which are high in blood pressure-deflating nutrients, rich in potassium, calcium, protein and fibre.

Dash also **discourages** foods that are high in saturated fats such as fatty meats, full fat dairy products and tropical oils, as well as sugar-sweetened beverages and sweets.

Most illnesses are due to the fact that our organs lack consistency and resistance. This is mostly because of a deficiency in minerals or trace elements. To remedy this, we need to eat enough vegetables.

CHAPTER TWO

WATER

Most of us can live without medicine, but no one can live without water. If everyone makes the best use of water, the amount of illnesses, especially in children, could be reduced.

The Ancient Greeks believed that there were four elements that God has used in creating everything that exists. The understanding of and mastery in the use of these four elements will definitely enable us to recreate ourselves and live sick-free to a grand old age. These four essential elements from which everything was made are: earth, air, water and fire.

We've already discussed much about air and earth elements. Let us now look at water. Water is the basis of all life forms. It was seen in the beginning as the origin of creation. Let us look at how water heals us at every level. Here are some examples:

The correct use of water is basic, in both the prevention and the treatment of diarrhoea. In many countries around the world, diarrhoea is the most common cause of illness and death in small children. Contaminated or unclean water is often part of the cause. Where water may be impure, an important part of the prevention of diarrhoea, is to boil or filter the water used for drinking or in the preparation of foods. A common cause of death in children with diarrhoea is severe dehydration, or the loss of too much water from the body. By giving a child with diarrhoea plenty of water, best with sugar or cereal salt, dehydration can often be prevented or corrected through rehydration.

Giving lots of liquids to a child with diarrhoea is more important than any medicine. In fact, if enough liquid is given, no medicine is usually needed in the treatment of diarrhoea.

There are many instances when the correct use of water may do more good than medicines. Here are some instances:

- To prevent skin infection, bathe often.
- To prevent wounds from becoming infected with tetanus, wash the wound well with soap and clean water in the morning, the afternoon and in the evening.
- To treat dehydration, drink plenty of liquids.
- For illnesses like fever drink plenty of water.
- Minor urinary infections that are common in women could be treated just by drinking plenty of water.
- To treat cough, asthma, bronchitis, pneumonia and whooping cough, drink plenty of warm water.
- Inflected wounds, abscesses and boils need hot soak or compresses.
- For stiff, sore muscles and joints, use hot compresses.
- For minor burns, hold in cold water at once.
- For strains and sprains, soak the joint in cold water on the first day, then use hot soaks subsequently.
- Use cold compresses for itching, burning or weeping irritations of the skin.
- For sore throat or tonsillitis, gargle with warm salty water.
- For acid, dye, dirt, or irritating substance in the eye, flush the eye with cold water at once, and continue for 30 minutes.
- To help stuffed up nose, sniff salty water.
- For constipation or hard stools, drink plenty of warm water.
- Enemas are also safer than laxatives, but do not overuse them.
- To treat cold sore or fever blister, hold ice on blister. For blisters in the palms, sock palm in warm water.

In each of the above cases, except pneumonia, when water is used correctly, medicines are often not required. Use medicines only when it is absolutely necessary.

Most people drink water the wrong way. When water is not drunk in the right way, it may be responsible for most shocking health problems like migraines, joint pains, skin problems, hair loss, digestive problems, heart pain, kidney problems, to name just a few. The sad part of it is that 98 percent of people usually drink water the wrong way, by which they unintentionally harm their bodies, rather than getting any benefits from this miraculous drink.

Without water our bodies cannot use the nutrients that come from carbohydrates, proteins and fats.

Because water is so essential to the functionality of the human body, it does not mean that we can drink water just about any way we want. Majority of people drink water immediately after a meal, which is very wrong. Drinking water immediately after meal is bad because it reduces the body's ability to digest food. Drink water mostly on an empty stomach. Drink water 30 minutes before meals and 30 minutes to one hour after meals.

Natural water is the best and safest medicine in the world. Drink 1 litre or 1.5 litres, normal or warm, first thing every morning, 1 litre at about noon, and another litre in the evening. Drink a little in between those intervals.

As you already know, water is indeed medicine. Drink it and drink it as long as you live, and not because you are thirsty, but because it's the rule and one of the best means to achieve a healthy long life. When you drink water when you are not thirsty, it acts like medicine. But when you drink when you are thirsty, it is food.

Whenever you start feeling tired, weak and sick during the day, or develop a headache, it is a sign that your blood and fluids are short of water, and so they are concentrated with toxins. Just get 1 to 1.5 litre of water and drink all of it.

Observe what happens a few minutes later. In addition to the water, breathe in deeply as previously explained, hold the breath for a few seconds and exhale slowly and deeply.

The Sensible Use of Medication

Here's valuable education about the sensible and limited usage of medication. Modern medicines are very important and do save lives. But for most ailments, no medication is required. The body itself can usually fight off diseases through the aid of the Positive and Negative Vital Life Energies.

Sometimes, someone may go to their doctor in hopes of receiving a prescription for medication, which they may not really need. Occasionally, the doctor may be tempted to prescribe some medication in order to satisfy a pestering patient. If they eventually feel better, they may believe that the medicines cured their ailments. However, instead of teaching people to depend on medication that they may not need, the doctor should, whenever necessary, explain to the patients why it should not be used.

It is important for people to know what they can do for themselves to get well. They need to know that there is no medicine that does not have some risk attached in its usage, and that the human body also has the capacity to heal itself.

There is something called over-medicalisation, by both doctors and the patients. This is unfortunate for many reasons, for it is not only wasteful, but it can create a dependency on drugs. Most money spent on medicines would be better spent on food. It makes people depend on something they do not need and often cannot afford. No medication is risk-free. There is always a chance that an unneeded medicine may actually cause harm to the body. What is more, when some medication is overused for minor problems, they lose their power to fight dangerous illnesses.

An example of medication that has lost its potency to heal is the over-prescribed antibiotic called Chloramphenicol.

The extreme overuse of this important drug means that in some parts of the world, it has lost its power to cure typhoid fever.

For all the above reasons the use of medication should be limited. Our bodies have their own defences, or ways to resist and fight off infection. In most cases, these natural defences are far more powerful to our health than any medicines. People will get well from most illnesses, including the common cold and the flu by themselves, without any need for medication.

To help the body fight off or overcome an illness, often all that is needed is to do enough deep breathing or enough exercises to inhale enough Positive Vital Life Energy, eat well and drink plenty of water, to obtain enough Negative Vital Life Energy. Keep the body clean and have plenty of rest. Even in cases of more serious illnesses, when a medication may be needed, it is usually the body that mostly overcomes the disease.

Natural Water and The Human Body

It should be noted that water accounts for 75% of the body's weight, that is, from 40 to 50 litres. It is spread throughout the body, in every one of our cells and between the cells. It circulates in the blood, the lymph glands, and in and around our organs. In fact, water safeguards the body in three main ways; the dissolution of nutrients and air elements, the purifying of waste and acids, the movement that allows for life and the renewal of tissue. Our bodies have constant need for repair and renewal which water makes possible.

Of its three functions, first and foremost, water is a purifying and cleansing agent.

- It dilutes acids, loosens waste and the used mineral salts that have given the body its magnetic strength, but are no longer useful.

- Water has the capacity to loosen the molecules that have to be secreted and transported away.
- It helps substances in the liver to change with the help of sulphur so that they can be removed.
- It ensures that acids can be secreted via the urine from the kidneys, and collects the trace elements (vitamins and minerals), depleted in magnetism. These reduce the energy value of the water so that it has to be removed from the body.

Another vital function of water is its ability to make things soluble.

- In this instance, it means water helps to break down nutrients in the body to facilitate their delivery to every cell.
- In fact, water enables the salts in the ground to penetrate the roots of plants, where its hydrogen molecules form organic molecules that our bodies can absorb.
- Water manufactures these molecules in our body that are able to renew tissue, make them fluid and soluble for transportation.

The third function of water is to allow the "spark of life" to manifest at the physical level because the incorporation of the spark of life in water brings about a fluid movement that has a continuous development in the cells. This makes growth and fertilisation possible.

Besides the assimilation we have discussed, these are the three most important phases of cellular life.

Bonded and free water: water is known to exhibit many physical properties in terms of the functionality we have just discussed above. We know that water in the body comes in two forms; it is either bonded to mineral salts, in particular, to sodium chloride which maintains its magnetic charge, or it exists in a free state not bonded by salts. In this case we can refer to it as pure or free water.

The water bonded by salts with its magnetic charge is called the Negative Polarity of Life. It strengthens the cohesion between our cells, restores our spirit and is concentrated in the cellular energy, which makes life possible to develop. What is special about bonded water is that it is a better conductor. It allows for the transmission of nerve influencing of the central nervous system.

Pure water (not bonded to salts) has another origin; it is free water. This water arises during cellular breathing. When the cells receive the oxygen from the blood, they become the carriers of the positive qualities of the life force. The oxygen along with the hydrogen of the nutrients is brought to the mitochondria (granular cells ranging from 0.5 to 1 micrometre in diameter,) which are the organs of the breathing cells. The nutrients consist of carbon and hydrogen molecules that carry the Negative Polarity of the Life Energy. Life is made possible by the joining of the hydrogen and oxygen, in that the two polarities of the Life Force are brought together. We could call this the Spark of Life. It involves the formation of new molecules of pure water. We can consider this pure intracellular water to be the assembly point of the divine consciousness, expressed as the Life Energy.

This water takes in the purity of the divine intelligence within itself and maintains it. The principle we discussed earlier is resolved here. The arrangement of the molecules and the elements become manifest and the hidden water principle is thus transmitted. Pure water is therefore not only useful in itself but useful for what it contains. When this feature of consciousness in the cell nucleus is expended, the water is no longer useful and it is excreted.

In summary, this water's energy brings its properties to the body. There, it recreates, revitalises, harmonises and restores human tissues, adding strength and capacity by passing this onto psychic strength. It supports the movement of life and contributes to a renewal of body tissues. In fact, the human body is actually made in the correct proportion of water, earth, fire and air. These four elements act within us in equal proportion through the four natural arrangements of these elements from the mind onwards, and from their harmony, our health hangs in the balance.

SLEEP AND REST

There are other factors which, if we are not vigilant, can cause disharmony in our bodies over a period of time. One of these factors is rest. We know that those who are in good health feel the greatest return of vigour after a good night's sleep. We also know that long-continuous decumbency or lying down; even with wakefulness, often follows a certain renewal of strength. An even greater renewal of vigour and vitality often follows a good sleep.

Whenever we feel exhausted by labour, sitting brings a partial return to vigour. It is also true that after the violent exertion of running, a lapse in the less violent exertion of walking, results in a gradual diminution of the troubling frustrations that the running had produced. Overwork can compromise the proper functioning of the human body, or what amounts approximately to the same thing as lack of rest.

It is therefore important for people to always remember that fatigue; no matter what form it takes, is an indication of an energy imbalance in the human body.

Overwork takes two forms: physical and intellectual exertions.

Physical overwork occurs most often during manual labour; involving tissues and muscular strengths of the human body. Any physical effort entails three major elements: an expenditure of energy, the death of certain types of cells and the secretion of various toxins. The best way to neutralise the effects these activities have on the human body is to sleep them off. It is mostly during sleep that the body compensates for its expenditure of energy, regenerates itself at the cellular level and eliminates a large number of toxins.

The second form of overwork is mental overwork, which usually arises from what would be called "intellectual" professions. The victims of these types of excesses are diverse. The consequences of mental overwork are more subtle than in the physical overwork. Any cerebral work still produces a loss of energy, but it is mostly at the level of the nervous system that its consequences are mostly marked. After a period of time, the individual involved will suffer from a loss of concentration, memory, reasoning, and cognition.

When a person is suffering from mental or physical overwork, the effects of such can be manifested in various forms, such as irritability, loss of appetite, depression, or even cardiovascular complications. In such cases, it is imperative to get some rest.

Our explanation regarding overwork now leads us to consider **sleep** and **rest**. It is common to hear someone say that they do not need to sleep or rest. But sleep, just like rest corresponds to a natural law. The cessation of activity is a necessary phase of human existence. Through an improper use of our free will, we may choose to ignore these laws, but we eventually pay within ourselves, by causing an energy imbalance, of which the consequences will be borne out in due course.

What is sleep? It is the period during which the voluntary functioning of the body is resting. On a mental level, it corresponds to the inactivity of the brain, or more exactly, to resting the purely objective phase of our consciousness. Sleep is also the regenerative processes of the body. During this period, the subconscious is completely free to work in the service of our body.

One in three of us suffer from poor sleeping habits. Usually, stress, computers and taking work home are often blamed.

However, the cost of all those sleepless nights is more than just bad moods and a lack of focus. Regular poor sleep puts the human body at risk of serious medical conditions, including obesity, diabetes and heart disease. It shortens one's life expectancy.

It is now clear that a solid night's sleep is essential for a long and healthy life. Most of us need about 8 hours of good quality sleep a night to function properly, but some need more and some even less. What matters is that you find out how much sleep you need and then try to achieve it every time. As a general rule, if you wake up tired and spend the day longing for a nap, then it is most likely that you are not getting enough sleep.

Fatigue, short temper and lack of focus often follow a poor night without sleep. An occasional night without sleep makes you feel tired and irritable the next day, but it won't harm you as several sleepless nights. After several sleepless nights, the mental effects become more severe. Your brain will fog, making it difficult to concentrate and make decisions. You'll start to feel down, and may fall asleep during the day. Your risk of injury and accidents at home, work and on the road also increases from lack of sleep.

If it continues, lack of sleep can affect your overall health and make you prone to serious medical conditions such as high blood pressure, diabetes, obesity and heart disease. Sleep boosts our immunity. If you seem to catch every cold and flu that's going around, it is possibly due to your sleeping habits or lack thereof. Prolonged lack of sleep can disrupt your immune system, so you are less able to fend off sicknesses.

Sleeping less can make you gain weight. Studies have shown that people who sleep less than 7 hours a day tend to gain more weight and stand a higher risk of becoming obese, than those who get 7 hours of proper sleep. It is believed that sleep-deprived people have reduced levels of leptin *(the chemical that makes one feel full)* and increased levels of ghrelin, *(the hunger stimulating hormone).*

Sleep prevents diabetes. Studies have suggested that people who usually sleep less than 5 hours a night have an increased risk of developing diabetes. It seems that missing out on deep sleep may lead to type 2 diabetes, by changing the way the body processes glucose, which the body uses for energy.

Sleep increase your sex drive. Men and women who do not get enough quality sleep have lower libidos and develop less of an interest in sex, research suggests. Men who suffer from sleep apnoea; a disorder in which breathing difficulties lead to interrupted sleep may also have lower libido.

Sleep increases fertility. It has been claimed that difficulties with conceiving a baby has been linked to the effects of sleep deprivation in both men and women. Apparently, regular sleep disruptions can cause trouble conceiving, by reducing the secretion of reproductive hormones.

Sleep wards off heart disease. Longstanding sleep deprivation seem to be associated with an increased heart rate, an increase in blood pressure and higher levels of certain chemicals linked with inflammation, which may put extra strain on the human heart.

Sleep boosts an overall mental wellbeing. Given that a single sleepless night can make you irritable and moody the following day, it is not surprising that chronic sleep deprivation may lead to long-term mood disorders like depression and anxiety. When people with anxiety or depression were surveyed to calculate their sleeping habits, it turned out that most of them slept for less than 6 hours a day.

THOUGHTS AND EMOTIONS

All illnesses are the result of one cause or another. Current medical practices tend to focus exclusively on one organ, or the physical part of the human body where the pain seems to originate, thus requiring treatment. Yet experience proves that the real causes of some diseases may not often located where the pain manifests. This means that treatment is generally worthless, if care is limited to a specific location for its origins without taking into consideration the general pathological condition of the person.

When the cause of an illness has been determined, it is necessary to eliminate the problem immediately, in order to help nature to re-establish harmony with the organ or the affected part of the body. At this point one may wish to resort to a therapeutic method for any personal choices.

We do have another effective means of harnessing the most favourable conditions within our own bodies in order to maintain good health. We are speaking of the curative powers of our thought. The thoughts we entertain have great influence on our physical wellbeing. That is why we recommend that you pay close attention to your mental attitude and what you're thinking about.

No treatment or therapy can result in the definitive healing of an illness, when its cause arises from poor mental hygiene—in other words, when a person habitually entertains negative thoughts. A person's health is not improved by merely thinking or wishing for good health. Rather, one must act in a concrete manner to turn their desires into a reality. In the realm of health, as well as in other areas, the famous maxim "God helps those who help themselves" still holds true.

Whether we are conscious of it or not, most of our thoughts give rise to our emotional state, for our psychological makeup is part of the whole human nature. Each emotion exerts a specific action on the autonomic nervous system, which directs and controls all the involuntary functions of the human body. This means that there is a constant interaction between our mental state and our general emotional state upon which the different centres charged with maintaining harmony in all its activities. When our emotional state is positive, such hormones or substances are secreted at rates consistent with the needs of the physical body and it contributes to its proper functioning.

On the other hand, when we are under the influence of negative emotions, these emotions also pour into our bloodstream in excessive quantities. Eventually, they give rise to a form of localised poisoning that temporally upsets some of the basic functioning of our organs. They also temporarily produce an increase in the circulatory flowing of the energy in the autonomic nervous system which negatively affects our general wellbeing.

Therefore, we must always try to keep ourselves in an emotional state that is as pure and positive as possible, so that we can vibrate in perfect resonance with the divine harmony.

An undeniable link exists between our mental and our emotional states. For example, when we are at peace with ourselves, our thoughts create harmony. If, on the other hand, we create inharmonious conditions; when we get angry or think selfish thoughts, our emotional state reflects our lack of harmony. On the other hand, beautiful or peaceful thoughts keep us relaxed and at peace.

Ugly thoughts can trigger ugly emotions. This leads to the third point; power that is destructive to our general wellbeing. In fact, many illnesses have their origins not only from external causes but within our own consciousnesses. Among the various fundamental causes of illness, it is important to mention the lack of inner harmony—or inner peace.

Far too many people lead lives based solely on earthly pleasures, even though they might not always realise this. By so doing, they completely neglect the most important dimensions of their being, and deprive themselves of that regenerative influx they could receive by acknowledging their own spirituality. If such people devoted as much attention to their spiritual selves as they do to their physical selves, they would be cured of most of the illnesses now afflicting them. They would raise their vibratory frequencies and remain in harmony with the divine.

We realise that such an assertion is unacceptable to many scientists but time will prove that physical, mental and spiritual harmony is the most effective of all cures. In fact, we are convinced that medicine will make its greatest strides when humanity becomes conscious of its divine nature and origins.

Our autonomic nervous system is extremely sensitive to the nature of our thoughts and emotions. The importance of the autonomic nervous system is often neglected by traditional medicine. This is a big mistake.

It is not unusual to hear someone say that an individual has recovered because he or she was in a “positive attitude”. Likewise, if another person succumbed to an illness, it could be because he or she had “a negative attitude”. When we are anxious, in anguish, or concentrating on negative thoughts; thoughts of hate and jealousy being the most destructive, we unconsciously disturb the whole system and lower the vibratory energy level of the nervous energy it distributes to all our organs. This disturbance causes a localised or a general loss of vitality.

Our nervous and muscular tension is likely intensified and manifests itself by violent gestures and words, which, of course, is in no way positive behaviour. In the fight to neutralise the excessive adrenaline which has poured into our blood stream, the body is forced to do extra unnecessary work and consequently it loses energy. This is a loss which could have been avoided and the energy put to more productive use.

Apart from the hormonal disorder they may produce, negative thoughts and emotions have a bad influence on such functions as breathing and digestion. For example, you are aware that we may experience considerable difficulty in breathing after an important psychological shock or a strong emotion. In such cases, the exchange of gases is abruptly interrupted, thus disturbing the equilibrium of the Vital Life Energy.

We truly hope that these explanations will enable you to understand the importance of your thoughts and emotions. Every time you allow yourself to slip into a disagreeable mental and emotional state, you affect your autonomic nervous system and its general functioning.

CHAPTER THREE

MEN'S HEALTH ISSUES

It is no myth to say that men's health has been greatly neglected and generally overlooked. This poses a danger that seems to be hiding in plain sight, nationally as well as globally. Great health for all cannot be achieved if the problems afflicting men are not addressed and well-managed.

This part of the writeup is aimed at putting invaluable information at your disposal to help men on their mission to achieve great health. There are cold hard facts to encourage you to trust and use the good techniques for balancing the Vital Life Force in your body. They will eventually spare you from the perils associated with an early grave, while you're able to live a healthy, disease-free existence to a ripe old age.

Here are some sobering facts with regards to men's health:

- Globally, the male life expectancy, at 68 years, lags five years behind the female life expectancy.
- There isn't a single country in the world in which male life expectancy exceeds that of the female.
- Overall, the gap between the sexes has increased since 1971 and will continue to widen if left unchecked.
- Men have a 40% probability of dying between the ages of 55 and 74, while in women, the probability is 30%.
- In over 80% of countries worldwide, the age-standardised death rate for cardiovascular disease is higher for men.
- In 2010, three times as many men as women died because of tobacco use.

- Almost one million more men than women died from dietary risk factors, such as low fruit and vegetable intake and from eating too many processed meats.
- Almost 90% of deaths attributable to occupational risk factors in 2010 were male. The two biggest occupational risks were injuries and exposure to particulate matter, gases and fumes.
- Men's health is problematic globally; and it is an issue that has so far been largely overlooked. It is about time this was systematically addressed on a national as well as on an international level.

Health policies and services have not always sought to engage with men. No wonder, the prevention of and the care for the health needs of men are noticeably absent in government and institutional policies. Unfortunately, the same problems associated with the neglect of men’s health needs are painfully apparent in the issues connected with the neglect of the health needs for boys.

Nevertheless, there are many reasons for seeking to improve men's health, besides it being an ethical and a moral imperative. Improvements in men’s health would reduce the burden on partners and children who depend on a man’s income or who could end up becoming their caregivers, to the detriment of their own income or education.

Men must make radical changes to balance the positive and negative polarities of the Vital Life Energies in their bodies, and ensure a commitment to a healthier diet, regular exercises and taking real rest. These are all tied to the best formulae for a healthy aging ritual. This pays dividends almost immediately one starts acting, and it is never too late to begin. A man who begins at 60 can live up to 85 years or even longer.

Understanding health risks is one thing, taking the necessary action to reduce those risks is another. Start by making healthy lifestyle changes. The impact might be greater than you ever imagined.

Staying healthy and preventing health problems are important ways to provide security for your family and your loved ones. So, take the necessary controls and learn what you can do now for yourself to obtain the best health in the years to come. Men's health issues are not as complicated as women's but with a healthy lifestyle, which includes regular exercising, eating healthy and not smoking, many major health risks that men face can be prevented.

ERECTILE DYSFUNCTION

Erectile dysfunction (ED) is one of the more common health issues older men face, especially those with cardiovascular diseases and diabetes. ED is defined as having difficulties in achieving or sustaining an erection. Some estimates suggest that between 50–70% of men; aged 50 and over, experience mild to moderate ED.

It is often caused by a combination of physical and emotional issues. ED makes intercourse difficult, which can lower the male sex drive and desire, increase anxiety and depression, and affect a man's relationship with his partner. Although it is more common in older men, ED can occur at any age.

The drugs to treat ED are standard solutions for most men, but they have their downsides, and other possible mild side effects, which includes a drug dependency habit. But pills should not be your first or only choice.

In many cases, lifestyle changes may slow the progress of ED and help manage it, so you may not need ED medications, or even be compelled to rely on them as much.

Remember we told you in chapter one that all diseases that have been diagnosed and catalogued are caused by a single fundamental cause; the lack of harmony or balance between the positive and negative polarities of the Vital Life Force in the body.

An analysis in the June 2018 issue of *Sexual Medicine* found that, on average, 40 minutes of moderate to vigorous aerobic activity, four times a week for six months, can improve ED. The type of exercise does not matter if the proper intensity is met. Examples include jogging, swimming, cycling, circuit-type resistance training, brisk walking, and deep breathing exercises. Diet and exercise go a long way to help restore a man's erection.

There are a couple of exercises you can do that will help towards achieving a healthier erection.

KEGEL EXERCISE

A Kegel exercise is done by tightening the muscles you would use to stop the flow of urine or to hold back gas. A typical routine consists of multiple Kegels with set amounts of time to hold the muscle contraction and to rest between repetitions. The number of reps can vary from 10 to 100 contractions. These exercises were developed in the late 1940s by Dr. Arnold H. Kegel, an American gynecologist, as a non-surgical way to prevent women from leaking urine. They also work for men who are plagued by incontinence.

Try performing Kegel exercises to strengthen your pelvic muscles. Some research suggests that, they may help with ED by increasing the blood flow to the penis.

How to Perform Kegel:

Women: Pretend you are trying to avoid passing out gas.

Pretend to tighten your vagina around a tampon.

Men: Pretend you are trying to avoid passing out gas.

While urinating, try to stop your urine stream.

Practice Contractions:

Choose your position.

Start by lying on your back until you get the feel of contracting the pelvic floor muscles.

When you have mastered it, practice while sitting and standing.

Contract and Relax

Contract your pelvic floor muscles for 4 to 6 seconds.
Relax for 4 to 6 seconds.
Repeat the contract-relax cycle 10 times.

Keep other muscles relaxed.

Don't contract your abdominal, leg, or buttocks muscles, or lift your pelvis.

Place a hand gently on your belly to detect unwanted abdominal action.

Extend the time

Gradually increase the length of contractions and relaxation.

Work your way up to 10 seconds contractions and relaxations.

Aim high

Try to do at least 30 to 40 Kegel exercises every day. Spreading them throughout the day is better than doing them all at once. Since these are stealth exercises that no one notices but you, try to sneak in a few when waiting at a stoplight, riding an elevator, or standing in a grocery line, etc.

Diversify:

Practice, 2 to 3 second contractions and releases (sometimes called "quick flicks") as well as longer ones.

Kegel exercises in an emergency

If you leak urine when you cough, sneeze, laugh, bend over,

or lift something heavy, doing one or more Kegels before a "trigger" may be enough to prevent any leakage.

Watch Your Waistline

A 2015 study found that clinically obese men have a 40% higher risk of developing ED. If you are overweight, reducing your weight by 5 to 10% has been shown to improve sexual function.

Change Your Diet

Several studies have found that the health benefits of a Mediterranean diet extend to ED too. See previous chapter that explains the Mediterranean diet.

ED can be red flag for other health issues like cardiovascular disease, diabetes, and prostate cancer.

Some Natural Herbs for ED Include:

- Coconuts and coconut water.
- Turmeric.
- Honey goat weed.
- Carrots.
- Ginger.
- Garlic.
- Beetroots.
- Banana.
- Roasted or fried plantains.
- Garri.
- Eggs.
- Salmon.
- Ashwagandha.
- Asparagus.
- Kaunch beej.
- Kali Musli.
- Shatavari.
- Maca roots amongst others.

TESTOSTERONE

Testosterone is the major sex hormone in males, and it plays several important roles, such as:

- The development of the penis and testes.
- The deepening of the voice during puberty.
- The appearance of facial and public hair starting at puberty; later in life, it may play a role in balding.
- Muscle size and strength.
- Bone growth and strength.
- Sex drive (libido) and sperm production.

Adolescent boys with too little testosterone may not experience normal masculinisation. For example, the genitals may not enlarge, facial and body hair may be scant, and the voice may not deepen normally.

If you thought testosterone was only important in men, you'd be mistaken. Testosterone is produced in the female ovaries and adrenal gland. It is one of several androgens (male sex hormones) in females.

These hormones are thought to have important effects on the following:

- Ovarian function.
- Bone strength.
- Sexual behaviour, including normal libido.

The proper balance between testosterone, (along with other androgens) and estrogen is important for the ovaries to work normally. While the specifics are uncertain, it's possible that androgens also play an important role in normal brain function (including mood, sex drive and cognitive function).

Testosterone is synthesised in the body from cholesterol. But having high cholesterol doesn't mean your testosterone will be high. Testosterone levels are too carefully controlled by the pituitary gland in the brain for that to occur.

The Perils of Too Much Testosterone

Having too much naturally occurring testosterone is not a common problem among men. That may not surprise you, given what people might consider obvious evidence of testosterone excess: fighting, aggressive, impatient, violence and sexual promiscuity is always associated with men. It is sometimes difficult to define "normal" testosterone levels. Blood levels of testosterone vary dramatically over time and even during the course of the day. In addition, what may seem like a symptom of testosterone excess may be unrelated to these hormones.

In fact, most of what we know about abnormally high testosterone levels in men comes from studying the actions of athletes, who use anabolic steroids, testosterone, or related hormones to increase muscles mass and athletic performance.

Problems associated with abnormally high testosterone levels in men include:

- Low sperm counts.
- Shrinking of the testicles and impotence.
- Heart muscle damage and increased risk of heart attack.
- Prostate enlargement with difficulty urinating.
- Fluid retention with swelling of the legs and the feet.
- Weight gain, perhaps related in part to increase appetite.
- High blood pressure and cholesterol.
- Increased muscle mass.
- Increased risk of blood clots.
- Stunted growth in adolescents.
- Uncharacteristically aggressive behaviour (although not well studied and clearly proven).
- Mood swings, euphoria, irritability, impaired judgment and delusion.
- Insomnia.

- Headache.
- Liver disease.
- Acne.

Among women, perhaps the most common cause of a high testosterone level is

Polycystic Ovary Syndrome (PCOS). This disease is common. It affects 6 - 10% of premenopausal women.

The ovaries of women with PCOS contain multiple cysts. Symptoms include irregular periods, reduced fertility, excess or coarse hair on the face, the extremities, the trunk and the pubic area, male-pattern baldness, thick skin, weight gain, depression, and anxiety. One treatment available for many of these problems is **Spironolactone**, a diuretic (water pill) that blocks the action of male sex hormones.

Women with high testosterone levels, due to either disease or drug use, may experience a decrease in their breast size and a deepening of their voice, in addition to many of the problems men may have.

Too Little Testosterone

In recent years, researches (and pharmaceutical companies) have focused on the effects of testosterone deficiency, especially among men. In fact, as men age, testosterone levels drop very gradually, about 1% to 2% each year, unlike the relatively rapid drop in estrogen that causes menopause. The testes produce less testosterone. More than a third of men over 45 years of age may a reduced level of testosterone than might be considered normal, (though, as mentioned, defining optimal levels of testosterone is tricky and somewhat controversial).

Symptoms of testosterone deficiency in adult males include:

- Reduced body and facial hair.
- Loss of muscle mass.

- Low libido, impotence, small testicles, reduced sperm count and fertility.
- Increased breast size.
- Irritability, poor concentration, and depression.
- Loss of body hair.
- Brittle bones and an increased risk of fracture.

Some men who have a testosterone deficiency, have symptoms or conditions related to their low testosterone that will improve when they have testosterone replacement. Regular negative breathing and deep positive breathing; together with a healthy balanced diet will help to keep the testosterone level in balance.

Did you know that there are times when low testosterone is not such a bad thing? The most common example is probably associated with prostate cancer. Testosterone may stimulate the prostate gland and prostate cancer to grow. That's why medications that lower testosterone levels (for example, Leuprolide) and castration are common treatments for men with prostate cancer. Men taking testosterone replacement must be carefully monitored for prostate cancer. Although testosterone may make prostate cancer grow, it is not clear that testosterone treatment actually causes cancer.

TREATMENT

The best testosterone treatment is AndroGel and Testim. It comes in packets of clear testosterone gel. It is absorbed directly through the skin when applied once a day. AndroGel, Axiron, and Fortesta also comes in a pump that delivers the amount of testosterone prescribed by your doctor.

Striant is a tablet that sticks to the upper gums above the incisors, the tooth just to the right or left of the two front teeth. Applied twice a day, it continuously releases testosterone into the blood through the tissues.

Injections and implants: testosterone can also be injected directly into the muscles, or implanted as pellets in the soft tissues.

Talk with your doctor about what is best for you.

Eating more vegetables can lower the risk of BPH. Green leafy vegetables are especially important because they are rich in antioxidants. Cruciferous vegetables such as broccoli also reduce the risk of prostate problems, including BPH and prostate cancer.

Avoid red meat, caffeine, alcohol, dairy products and sodium. In addition to eating a healthy diet, you should stay active. Regular exercise pares down the risk of developing some deadly problems including heart disease, stroke, and certain types of cancer.

PROSTATE

The prostate is a gland that is a part of the male reproductive system that wraps around the male urethra near the bladder. The gland is about the size of a walnut and grows larger as you age. Enlargement of the prostate gland can cause symptoms such as:

- Dribbling urine.
- Pain or burning during urination.
- Frequent urination.
- Blood in the seamen or urine.
- Frequent pain or stiffness in the lower back, hips, pelvic, or rectal area or the upper thighs.
- Urination incontinence (the inability to urinate).
- And painful ejaculation.

Common Prostate Problems in Men Include:

- Benign prostatic hyperplasia.
- Acute and chronic bacteria prostatitis.
- Chronic Prostatitis (non-bacteria).

PROSTATE CANCER

Treatment for prostate cancer depends on whether the cancer is in part or all of the prostate or if it has spread (metastasised) to other parts of the body. It also depends on your age and overall health. For cancer that has not spread from the prostate to other parts of the body, your doctor may suggest:

- Watchful waiting or active surveillance. If the cancer is growing slowly and not causing problems, you may not to treat it right away. Instead regularly infuse yourself with the Power of Life (the positive and negative polarity of the Vital Life Forces) through deep breathing exercises and proper dieting. While infusing your body with the Power of Life (the Vital Life Force), your doctor will check regularly for changes in your condition.
- Surgery. The most common type of surgery removes the whole prostate and some nearby tissue.
- Radiation therapy. This treatment uses radiation to kill cancer cells and shrink tumors.
- Hormone therapy. Men having other treatments like radiation therapy may also be treated with drugs to stop the body from making testosterone.

STROKES

A stroke occurs when a blockage or bleed of the blood vessels either interrupts or reduces the supply of blood to the brain. When this happens, the brain does not receive enough Positive Vital Life Force in the oxygen or the Negative Vital Life Energy from nutrients, and the brain cells start to die. Some studies have found that males have a higher risk of death from stroke than females.

A stroke is also a cerebrovascular disease. This means that it affects the blood vessels that feed the oxygen to the brain.

If the brain does not receive enough oxygen, damage may start to occur.

SYMPTOMS

The symptoms of a stroke often appear without warning. Some of the main symptoms include:

- Confusion, including difficulty speaking and understanding speech.
- A headache, possibly with altered consciousness or vomiting.
- Numbness or an inability to move parts of the face, arm, or legs, particularly on one side of the body.
- Vision problems in one or both eyes.
- Difficulty walking, including dizziness and a lack of coordination.

A stroke can lead to long-term health problems. Depending on the speed of the diagnosis and treatment, a person can experience temporary or permanent disabilities after a stroke.

Causes and Risk Factors

Each type of stroke has a different set of potential causes. Generally, however, a stroke is more likely to affect a person if the following conditions are present:

- There is an imbalance or lack of equilibrium of the positive and negative polarity of the Vital Life Energies in the body.
- Have heart disease, carotid artery disease, or another vascular disease.
- Smoke, consume alcohol excessively, use illicit drugs or are sedentary.
- Have overweight or obesity.
- Are 55 years of age or older.
- Have a personal or family history of stroke.
- Have high blood pressure.

- Have high cholesterol or diabetes.

Prevention

- Exercise regularly, to obtain enough positive vitality of the Vital Life Force.
- Eat a healthy diet and drink enough water to obtain enough polarity of the Negative Vital Life Energy.
- Avoid alcohol, or only drink moderately.
- Don’t smoke tobacco.
- Maintain a moderate weight.

ALZHEIMER'S DISEASE

Alzheimer's disease is an irreversible, progressive brain disorder that slowly destroys memory and thinking skills, and, eventually, the ability to carry out the simplest tasks. In most people with Alzheimer's, symptoms first appear in their mid-60s.

Alzheimer's disease is currently ranked as the sixth leading cause of death in the United States, but recent estimates indicate that the disorder may rank third, just behind heart disease and cancer, as a cause of death for older people. Alzheimer's is the most common cause of dementia among older adults. Dementia is the lost of cognitive functioning—thinking, remembering, and reasoning-and behavioural abilities to such an extent that it interferes with a person's daily life and activities. Dementia ranges in severity from the mildest stage, when it is just beginning to affect a person's functioning, to the most serve stages, when the person must depend completely on others for basic activities of daily living.

Causes of Alzheimer's Disease

Scientists don't yet fully understand what causes Alzheimer's in most people. But as you are already aware, the cause of all sickness is an imbalance of the positive and negative polarity of the Vital Life Energies in the body. The causes probably include a combination of genetic, environmental, and lifestyle factors.

Common behavioural symptoms of Alzheimer's include sleeplessness, wandering, agitation, anxiety, and aggression.

Prevention

We already know that for a natural healthy life to exist, there must be a balanced combination of the Positive and Negative Vital Life Energies. A nutritious diet, physical activity, social engagement, and mentally stimulating pursuits have all been associated with helping people stay healthy as they age.

CHRONIC OBSTRUCTIVE PULMONARY DISEASE

Chronic obstructive pulmonary disease (COPD) is a chronic inflammatory lung disease that causes obstructive airflow from the lungs. Symptoms include breathing difficulties, cough, mucus, (sputum) production and wheezing. It is typically caused by long-term exposure to irritating gases or particulate matter—most often from cigarette smoke. People with (COPD) are at increased risk of developing heart disease, lung cancer, and a variety of other conditions.

Symptoms

COPD symptoms often don't appear until significant lung damage has occurred, and they usually worsen over time, particularly if smoking exposure continues.

Signs and symptoms may include:

- Shortness of breath, especially during physical activities.
- Wheezing; chest tightness.
- A chronic cough that may produce mucus (sputum) that may be clear, white, yellow or greenish.

- Frequent respiratory infections.
- Lack of energy.
- Unintended weight loss.
- Swelling in ankles, feet or legs.

Causes

The main cause of COPD in developed countries is tobacco smoking. In the developing world, COPD often occurs in people exposed to fumes from burning fuel for cooking and heating in poorly ventilated homes. Only some chronic smokers develop clinically apparent COPD, although many smokers with long smoking history may develop reduced lung function. Some smokers develop less common lung conditions. They may be misdiagnosed as having COPD until a more thorough evaluation is performed.

Prevention

Unlike some diseases, COPD typically has a clear cause and a clear path to prevention. The majority of cases are directly related to cigarette smoking, and the best way to prevent it is to never smoke, or to stop smoking now. If you're a long-time smoker, these simple statements may not seem so simple, especially if you tried quitting once, twice or many times before. But keep trying to quit. It is your best chance for reducing damage to your lungs.

Occupational exposure to chemical fumes and dusts is another risk factor for COPD. If you work with these types of lung irritants, talk to your supervisor about the best ways to protect yourself, such as using respiratory protective equipment.

Get an annual flu vaccination and regular vaccination against pneumococcal pneumonia to reduce your risk of or prevention of some infections.

RECIPE FOR SMOKERS

If you smoke, or even if you have smoked for 5 years and above, this recipe will easily clear your lungs. Smoking is a harmful habit that puts your health in danger. It has negative influence on the whole human body, but the lungs are the front line.

Ingredients:

You will need a glass of honey
2 teaspoons of turmeric powder
1 ginger root
400g garlic

Preparation:

Peel and chop the turmeric, ginger and garlic. Add all these ingredients in a litre of water and boil for five minutes. Let it cool at room temperature. Keep this mixture in the refrigerator.

Take 2 tablespoons on an empty stomach every morning before breakfast and in the evening a few hours after dinner.

Cleansing the Lungs Needs Time and Patience.

How to Detoxify the Lungs

Here is another powerful lungs cleanser.

Blend 3 roots of carrots, half a cup of lemon juice, and a litre of water. Boil for 5 minutes. Cool it down. Add some honey. Keep it in the refrigerator. Take 2 tablespoons, full 3 times a day: morning, afternoon, and evening.

LIVER DISEASE

Your liver is an important organ that performs hundreds of tasks related to your metabolism, energy storage, and detoxification of waste. It helps to digest food, convert it to energy, and store the energy until you need it. It also helps filter toxic substances out of your bloodstream. Anything keeping your liver from doing its job puts your life in danger. It's every man's duty to use the Vital Life Energies to maintain a natural healthy liver. A healthy liver has the amazing ability to grow back, regenerate when damaged.

Causes of Liver Disease

Liver disease has many causes.

Infection: Parasites and viruses can infect the liver, causing inflammation that reduces liver function. The viruses that cause liver damage can be spread through blood or semen, contaminated food or water, or close contact with a person who is infected. The most common types of liver infections are hepatitis A, B and C. Immune system abnormality diseases in which your immune system attacks certain parts of your body (autoimmune) can affect your liver.

Genetics

An abnormal gene inherited from one or both of your parents can cause various substances to build up in your liver causing liver damage.

Cancers

Examples include:

Liver cancer; Bile duct cancer and liver adenoma.

Other Causes

Additional, common causes of liver disease include:

- Chronic alcohol abuse.
- Fat accumulation into the liver.
- Certain prescription or over-the-counter medications.
- Certain herbal compounds such as ma Huang and kava kava. The plant ephedra (ma Huang) contains multiple chemical compounds, but the most notable is ephedrine. This molecule impacts several bodily

processes and was used as a popular dietary supplement ingredient prior to being banned in several countries.

Kava is a tropical evergreen shrub with heart-shaped leaves. The roots of the kava plant contain compounds call kava lactones. The current research supports the use of kava for treating anxiety. It tends to be as effective as certain anxiety drugs, with no evidence of dependency. Though kava can be used safely in the short term, it has been linked to liver problems.

Other Risk Factors

Factors that may increase the risk of Liver disease include:

- Obesity.
- Type 2 diabetes.
- Tattoo or body piercing.
- Injecting drugs using shared needles.
- Exposure to other people's blood and body fluids.
- Unprotected sex.
- Exposure to certain chemicals or toxins.
- A family history of liver disease.
- Imbalance of the positive and negative polarities of the Vital Life Forces.

Prevention

- Drink alcohol in moderation.
- Avoid risky behaviour. Use a condom during sex.
- If you choose to have tattoos or body piercings, be picky about cleanliness and safety when selecting a shop.
- Seek help if you use illicit intravenous drugs, and don't share needles to inject drugs.
- Get vaccinated. If you are at increased risk of contracting hepatitis or if you've already been infected with any form of the hepatitis virus, talk to

your doctor about getting the hepatitis A and B vaccines.

- Use medications wisely. Take prescription and non-prescription drugs only when needed and only in recommended doses. Don't mix medications and alcohol.
- Avoid contact with other people's blood and body fluids.
- Keep your food and water safe.
- Take care with aerosol sprays. Make sure to use these products in a well - ventilated area, and wear a mask when spraying insecticides, fungicides, paint and other toxic chemicals. When using insecticides and other toxic chemicals, wear gloves, long sleeves, a hat and a mask so that chemicals aren't absorbed through your skin.
- Maintain a healthy weight.

How to Detoxify Your Liver

You will need a handful of fresh lemongrass or mint leaves, orange, lemon, organic honey and one litre of water.

Preparation:

Pour a litre of water a pot. Turn on the stove and bring the water to a boil for 5 minutes. Turn off the stove. Put the lemon grass and orange juice inside along with the grated lemon. Add some honey to taste. You can consume this drink hot or cold. Take a glass morning and evening, every day for one week, then take a pause and repeat it whenever you think it is necessary.

DIABETES

Diabetes mellitus, commonly known as diabetes, is a metabolic disease that causes high blood sugar. With diabetes, your body either doesn't make enough insulin or can't effectively use the insulin it makes. Untreated high blood sugar from diabetes can damage the nerves, eyes, kidneys, and other organs.

The most common types of diabetes are:

Type 2 diabetes. A chronic condition that affects the way the body processes blood sugar (glucose).

Type 1 diabetes. A chronic condition in which the pancreas produces little or no insulin.

Prediabetes. A condition in which blood sugar is high, but not high enough to be type 2 diabetes.

Causes of Diabetes.

Prediabetes: It is caused by an imbalance of the Positive and Negative Vital Life Energies in the body.

Type 1 diabetes: Doctors don't know exactly what causes type 1 diabetes. For some reason, the immune system mistakenly attacks and destroys insulin in the body, which results in the production of beta cells in the immune system. What weakens the immune system is an imbalance of the Vital Life Force in the body.

Type 2 diabetes: It stems from a combination of genetics and lifestyle factors. Being overweight or obese increases the risk too.

Symptoms

The general symptoms include:

- Increased hunger.
- Increased thirst.

- Weight loss.
- Frequent urination.
- Blurred vision.
- Extreme fatigue.
- Sores that don't heal.

Symptoms in Men:

In addition to the general symptoms of diabetes, men with diabetes may have a decrease in their sex drive, erectile dysfunction (ED), and poor muscle strength.

Symptoms in Women:

Women can also have symptoms such as urinary tract infections, yeast, and dry itchy skin.

Prevention

Remember that all diseases that have been diagnosed and catalogued are caused by a single fundamental cause, lack of harmonium. If there is a lack of balance between the Positive and Negative Vital Life Energies in the body, it will create a lack of harmony in the entire organism and decrease the vibratory frequency of the body. This causes all types of illnesses, including diabetes, liver problems, kidney diseases, stroke, cancer, heart disease, prostate, testosterone, blood pressure, gynecological problems, depression, and anxiety. He who is aware of this great law or principle of balance will never stray from its equilibrium.

Type 1 diabetes is caused by a problem in the immune system. Its only preventive measure is to maintain a balance of the Vital Life energy in the body. Most diabetes-prevention strategies involve making simple adjustments to your diet and fitness routine.

If you have been diagnosed with prediabetes, here are a few things you can do to delay or prevent type 2 diabetes:

- Get at least 150 minutes per week of aerobic exercise, such as walking, or cycling.
- Cut saturated and trans fats, along with refined carbohydrate, out of your diet.
- Eat more fruits, vegetables and whole grains.
- Eat smaller portions.
- Try to lose 7% of your bodyweight if you're overweight or obese.
- Drink water as your primary beverage.
- Quit smoking.
- Follow a very low carb diet.
- Eat a diet that's rich in fibre.
- Optimise your vitamin D levels.
- Minimise your intake of processed foods.
- Drink coffee or tea.

Natural Herbs

Curcumin and Berberine. These herbs increase insulin sensitivity, reduce blood sugar levels and may help prevent diabetes.

KIDNEY DISEASE

Healthy kidneys are essential to having a healthy body. They are mainly responsible for filtering waste products, excess water, and other impurities out of the bloodstream. These toxins are stored in the bladder and then removed during urination. The kidneys also regulate PH, salt, and potassium levels in the body. They produce hormones that regulate the blood pressure and control the reproduction of red blood cells. The kidneys even activate a form of vitamin D that helps the body to absorb calcium.

Kidney disease occurs when the kidneys become damaged and cannot perform their functions normally. Damage may be caused by an imbalance of the Vital Life Energy in the body, diabetes, high blood pressure, and various other chronic (long-term) conditions. Kidney disease can lead to other health problems, including weak bones, nerve damage, and malnutrition.

If the disease gets worse over time, the kidneys may stop working completely. This means that dialysis will be required to perform the function of the kidneys. Dialysis is a treatment that filters and purifies the blood using a machine. It can't cure kidney disease, but it can prolong life.

Symptoms of Kidney Disease

Kidney disease is a condition that can easily go unnoticed until the symptoms become severe. The following *symptoms are early warning signs* that one might be developing kidney disease.

- Fatigue.
- Difficulty concentrating.
- Trouble sleeping.
- Poor appetite.
- Muscle cramping.
- Swollen feet and ankles.
- Puffiness around the eyes in the morning.
- Dry scaly skin.
- Frequent urination especially late at night.

Severe symptoms that could mean a kidney disease progressing into kidney failure include:

- Nausea.
- Vomiting.
- Loss of appetite.
- Changes in urine output.
- Fluid retention.
- Anemia.
- Decreased sex drive.
- Sudden rise in potassium levels (hyperkalemia).
- Inflammation of the pericardium (fluid-filled sac that covers the heart).

Prevention

Some risk factors for kidney disease such as age, race, or family history, are impossible to control. However, there are measures you can take to help prevent kidney disease:

- Drink plenty of water.
- Control blood sugar if you have diabetes.
- Control blood pressure.
- Reduce salt intake.
- Quit smoking.

Over-the-counter drugs

You should always follow the dosage instructions for over-the-counter medications. Taking too much aspirin, (Bayer) or ibuprofen (Advil, Motrin) can cause kidney damage.

Limit certain foods.

Different chemicals in your food can contribute to certain types of kidney stones.

These include:

Excessive sodium.

Animals protein, such as beef and chicken.

Citric acid, found in citrus fruits such as oranges, lemons, and grapefruits.

Oxalate; a chemical found in beets, spinach, sweet potatoes, and chocolate.

Foods to add to your diet

Berries; such as strawberries and blueberries, apples; grapefruits; pineapples, cauliflower; broccoli; eggplant; green beans; white rice; white pasta; white bread; egg whites.

Foods to limit or avoid when one has kidney disease.

- Bananas
- Avocados
- Raisins
- Prunes and prunes juice
- Tomatoes, tomato juice and tomato sauce
- Lentils
- Spinach
- Brussels sprouts
- Split pears
- Potatoes (regular and sweat)
- Pumpkin
- Dried apricots
- Milk
- Bran products
- Low-sodium cheese
- Nuts
- Beef and chicken

HOW TO DETOXIFY THE KIDNEYS NATURALLY:

Beetroots: The benefits of beetroot include the fact that it has anti-cancer and antioxidants properties. It also amplifies the greatness of urine.

Watermelon juice: It is composed of 92% of water. It can help in melting the kidney stones and trash too.

Celery: Celery contains properties that aid in removing toxins from the body by increasing urination. Regular intake can prevent kidney stones and infections.

Ginger: It helps flush harmful toxins out of the kidneys and improves digestion. This herb is beneficial for cleansing the liver.

Corn silk: It can be used to treat bladder infections, kidney stones and urinary infections.

Parsley: Parsley promotes increased urine output to help flush bacteria and germs out of the kidneys.

CANCERS

Cancer is a group of diseases involving abnormal cell growth, with the potential to invade or spread to other parts of the body. These contrast with benign tumors, which do not spread. Cancer is a broad term. It describes the disease that results when cellular changes cause the uncontrolled growth and division of cells. Some types of cancers cause rapid cell growth, while others cause cells to grow and divide at a slower rate.

Certain forms of cancer result in visible growths called tumors, while others, such as leukemia do not. Most of the body's cells have specific functions and fixed lifespans. While it may sound like a bad thing, cell death is part of a natural and beneficial phenomenon called *apoptosis.* In normal body functioning, a cell receives instructions to die so that the body can replace it with a newer cell that functions better. Cancerous cells lack the components of *apoptosis* that instruct them to stop dividing and to die. As a result, they build up in the body, using oxygen and nutrients that would usually nourish other cells. Cancerous cells can form tumors, impair the immune system and cause other changes that prevent the body from functioning regularly. Cancerous cells may appear in one area, then spread via the lymph nodes. These are clusters of immune cells located throughout the body.

CAUSES

There are many causes of cancer, and some are preventable. For example, over 480,000 people die in the US each year from cigarette-smoking-related cancers, according to data reported in 2014.

In addition to smoking, risk factors for cancer include:

- An imbalance of the positive and negative polarity of the Vital Life Energies in the body.
- Heavy alcohol consumption.
- Physical inactivity.
- Poor nutrition.
- Aging.
- Genetic.

Treatment

Innovative research has fueled the development of new medications and treatment technologies for many types of cancers. Doctors usually prescribe treatments based on the type of cancer, its stage at diagnosis, and the person's overall health.

Below are examples of approaches to cancer treatment:

Deep Breathing and Diet.

A balance between the positive and negative polarities of the Vital Life Force in the body through deep breathing and nutrition is the most important step to begin treatment, while on medication. Almost every physician suggests that a balanced diet and good nutrition and enough exercise will help an individual combat cancer or any disease.

- Chemotherapy aims to kill cancerous cells with medications that target rapidly dividing cells. The drugs can also help shrink tumors, but the side effects can be severe.
- Hormone therapy.
- Immunotherapy.
- Radiation therapy.
- Stem cell.
- Surgery.

Doctors often employ more than one type of treatment to maximise effectiveness.

Home Remedies

There are many claims on the internet and in publications about substances that treat cancer. For example, broccoli, grapes, ginseng, soybeans, green tea, aloe vera, garlic, turmeric, carrots, blueberries, papaya and treatments like acupuncture, vitamins, and dietary supplements.

Patients are strongly recommended to discuss any home remedies or alternative treatments with their cancer doctors before beginning any of these.

Prevention

- Never ever forget that, for a natural healthy life to exist, there must be a balanced combination of the positive and negative polarities of the Vital Life Forces in the body. To live in this balance is the first step to preventing cancer or any disease.
- Stop or better still, never start smoking tobacco.
- Avoiding excess sunlight (by decreasing exposure or applying sunscreens).
- Avoiding many chemicals and toxins is an excellent way to avoid cancers.
- Avoiding contact with certain viruses and other pathogens also are likely ways to prevent some cancers.
- Maintain a healthy weight and be physically active.
- Practice safe sex and avoid risky behaviours.
- Get immunization (HPV and Hepatitis vaccines).

CHAPTER 4

WOMEN'S HEALTH

With healthcare, some problems are universal but there are other health-related issues that are gender specific; and may only affect one sex. Other times, certain health needs affect females at a higher rate than males or vice versa.

The first step to understanding female health needs is education. Many women are simply unaware of the risk factors that lead to serious health problems, and they miss out on valuable opportunities that they could take to minimize the associated dangers. While some risk factors are genetic, others are based on lifestyles.

The first and the most important step to take is to get more information. With regards to personal health, knowledge is a powerful tool in the hands of every individual. The more you know about the risk factors associated with your health, the easier and the better off you are on how to manage them. When it comes to building a healthy community, the importance of health education cannot be overestimated.

There are many health problems prevalent with women's health: but the ones which pose the greatest threats are the following:

- Heart disease
- Breast cancer
- Ovarian and Cervical cancer
- Gynecological health
- Pregnancy-related issues
- Autoimmune diseases
- Depression
- Anxiety and stress
- Diabetes
- High Blood pressure

- Sexually transmitted diseases or STDs

HEART DISEASE

Heart disease is the leading killer for both men and women, but most women tend to be underdiagnosed to the point where it is too late to help them, once the condition is discovered. Many studies suggest that in women, the symptoms may not just be chest pain. Symptoms like jaw pain, shoulder pain, nausea, or shortness of breath should also be considered.

Women can reduce their risk of heart disease by modifying their lifestyles to include a well-balanced diet, and exercise to enable them to have a good balance of the Vital Life Force (VLF) in the body.

HOW TO NATURALLY IMPROVE A HEALTHY HEART

For most of us, preventing heart disease depends largely on our lifestyles, which means there's much that's in our power to improve the odds of us living long and well. The use of medications; where appropriate, can be beneficial, but medications should be adjunct to lifestyle improvements like healthy foods and exercise, to enable us to balance the Vital Life Force in the human body.

Diet and exercise have been proven to:

- Dramatically reduce heart disease risk factors.
- Stabilize plaques in the arteries so they are less likely to burst and trigger blood clots that block blood flow, causing heart attacks.
- Reverse the progression of coronary artery disease or atherosclerosis.
- In decades past, physicians were trained in the diagnosis and treatment of coronary artery disease after it occurred.

However, the present epidemic of cardiovascular diseases, diabetes, and their complications of heart attack, stroke, heart failure, and sudden death have necessitated a change of focus to prevention. What we can achieve, from a natural lifestyle-based approach has no drug substance.

Change is an important part of living with heart disease or trying to prevent it. Heart attack and stroke survivors are often told to alter a lifetime of habits.

Some people manage to overhaul their exercise pattern, diet, and unhealthy habits with ease. The rest of us try to make changes, but don't always succeed. Instead of undertaking a huge makeup, you might be able to improve your heart's health with a series of small changes. Once you get going, you may find that change isn't so hard. This approach may take longer, but it could also motivate you to make some big changes.

Here are some small steps to improve the heart.

- Take a 10-minutes’ walk. If you don't exercise at all, a brief walk is a way to start. If you do, it's a good way to add exercise to your day.
- Do some lifts. Lifting a hardcover book or a two pounds weight a few times a day can help tone your arm muscle. When that becomes easy, move on to heavier items or join a gym.
- Eat one extra fruit or vegetable a day. Fruits and vegetables are inexpensive, taste good and are good for everything, from your brain to your bowels.
- Make breakfast count. Start the day with some fruits and serving of whole grains, like oatmeal, bran flakes, or whole-wheat toast.
- Cutting out one sugar sweetened soda or calorie-laden latte can easily save you 100 or more calories a day. Over a year, that can translate into a 10-pound weight loss.

- Have a handful of nuts. Walnuts almonds, peanuts and other nuts are good for your heart.
- Sample the fruits of the sea. Eat fish or other types of sea food, instead of red meat once a week. It is good for the heart, the brain and the waistline.
- Breathe deeply. Remember that to obtain enough Positive Vital Life Energy in the body, we need deep breathing. Try breathing slowly and deeply for a few minutes a day. It can help you relax. Slow, deep breathing may also help to lower blood pressure.
- Wash your hands often. Scrubbing up with soap and water often during the day is a great way to protect your heart and health. The flu, pneumonia, and other infections can be very hard on the health.
- Taking a moment each day to acknowledge the blessings in your life is one way to start tapping into other positive emotions. These have been linked with better health, long life, and greater wellbeing, just as their opposites, chronic anger, worry, and hostility, contribute to high blood pressure and heart disease.

CARDIAC MEDICATIONS

Once an individual has suffered a heart attack, that person will most likely be prescribed medications that they will take for the rest of their life. Here are some of the major types of commonly prescribed cardiovascular medications to serve as guides. However, we're not recommending or endorsing any specific products. If your prescription medication is not on the list, remember that your healthcare provider and pharmacists are your best sources of information. It is important to discuss all the drugs you take with your doctor and understand their desired and possible side effects. Never stop taking a medication and never change your dose without first consulting the prescribing doctor.

- Anticoagulants.
- Antiplatelet Agents and Dual.

- Antiplatelet Therapy.
- ACE Inhibitors.
- Angiotensin 11 Receptor Blockers.
- Angiotensin Receptor-Neprilysin Inhibitors.
- Beta Blocker.
- Calcium Channel Blockers.
- Cholesterol-lowering medications.
- Digital preparation.
- Diuretics.
- Vasodilators.

BREAST CANCER

We are on a mission to get rid of illnesses and free the world from sickness and pain, by spreading the word on prevention, so that you can live longer and better. One perennial problem affecting women's health is breast cancer. Raising the public awareness for breast cancer is a key strategy to control the disease. Youth and young adult years are key times for helping to prevent breast cancer in life. Healthy behaviours started in youth and continued throughout life can prevent 60 percent or more of all breast cancers.

It is never too early or late to get started with a healthy lifestyle, and this is especially true when it comes to breast cancer. Research shows that lifestyle changes can decrease the risk of breast cancer, even in women at high risk.

The following can help lower the risks associated with breast cancer:

Be Physically Active

Women who are physically active for at least 30 minutes a day have a lower risk of breast cancer. Regular exercise is also one of the best ways to help increase the positive polarity of the Vital Life Force in the body, which helps to prevent many pathological illnesses.

Diet

A healthy diet can help lower the risks of breast cancer. Try to eat a lot of fruits and vegetables and keep alcohol at moderate levels or lower. While moderate drinking can be good for the heart in older adults, even low levels of intake can increase the risks of breast cancer. If you don't drink, don't feel you need to start. If you drink moderately, there's likely no reason to stop. But if you drink more, then you should cut down or quit.

Eating a healthy diet might decrease your risks of cancer as well as diabetes, heart disease and stroke. For example, women who eat a Mediterranean diet have a reduced risk of breast cancer. (*Refer to Mediterranean diet in earlier parts of this writeup)*

Don't Smoke

Smokers and non-smokers alike know how unhealthy smoking is. On top of lowering the quality of the Positive Vital Life Force, thus lowering the quality of life and increasing the risk of heart disease, stroke and at least 15 cancers, including breast cancer, it also causes smelly breath, bad teeth, and wrinkles. Now that's motivation to stay smoke free or work to get out of it.

Breastfeed Where Possible

Breastfeeding for a total of one year or more lowers the risks of breast cancer. It also has great health benefits for the child.

Birth Control Pills

Avoid birth control pills, especially after the age of 35 or if you are a smoker. Birth control pills have both risks and benefits. The younger a woman is, the lower the risks are. Women who are taking birth control pills have a slightly increased risk of breast cancer. This risk goes away quickly after stopping the pills. The risk of stroke and heart attack is also increased while on the pills, especially if the woman is a smoker. However, long-term use can also have important benefits; like lowering the risks of ovarian cancer, colon cancer and uterine cancer—not to mention unwanted pregnancy. So, there is also a lot in its favour but if you're worried about contracting breast cancer, avoiding birth control pills is one option to help lower the risks.

Avoid Menopausal Hormone Therapy

Menopausal hormone therapy shouldn't be taken long term, in order to avoid chronic diseases like Osteoporosis and heart disease. Studies show that it has a mixed effect on health, increasing the risk of some diseases and lowering the risks of others. Both estrogen-only hormones and estrogen-plus-progestin hormones increase the risks of breast cancer.

If women do take menopausal hormone therapy, it should be for the shortest time possible. The best person to talk to about the risks and benefits of menopausal hormone therapy is your doctor.

Tamoxifen and Raloxifene

Although not commonly thought of as a "healthy behaviour" taking the prescription drugs tamoxifen and raloxifene can significantly lower the risks of breast cancer in women at high risk of the disease. These powerful drugs can have side effects, so they aren't right for everyone. If you think you are at high risk, talk to your doctor to see if tamoxifen and raloxifene may be right for you.

OTHER IMPORTANT RISK FACTORS

Unfortunately, there are also several important breast cancer risk factors that women have no control over. Knowing which one applies to you can help you to understand your risk and do what you can to lower it.

- Old age, especially 60 years or over
- Family history of breast cancer (genetic factors)

- Early menopausal period (menarche) before age 12
- Menopause aged 55 or over
- First childbirth after the age of 35
- No children (never conceived)
- Tall height (5' 8" or taller)
- Dense breasts
- History of benign breast cancer (like atypical hyperplasia)

Don't Forget Screening

Despite some controversy, studies show that breast cancer screening, with mammography saves lives. It doesn't help prevent cancer, but it can help to detect cancer in its early stages when it is most treatable.

CERVICAL DYSPLASIA

Cervical dysplasia is a precancerous condition of the cervix caused by the human papilloma virus (HPV). Cervical dysplasia usually appears without symptoms. Therefore, it is advisable to see your doctor for an annual examination, as well as for regular pap smears after the age of 21, to screen for any abnormal cells.

Cervical Dysplasia Treatment

For both moderate and severe cases of cervical dysplasia, a loop electrosurgical excision procedure (LEEP,) to biopsy the cervical tissue may be recommended.

Patients ages 9 to 26 can receive an HPV vaccine to protect against the four most common strains of the virus. The recommended age is between 9 and 11 before your child becomes sexually active, and both boys and girls can receive the vaccine.

MENSTRUAL DISORDERS

Heavy or prolonged menstrual bleeding, bleeding during intercourse, bleeding between periods and especially painful cramps can be signs of a menstrual disorder in women of menstruating age. Depending on the menstrual cycle problem or condition and the severity, medical and/or surgical intervention methods are available.

Menstrual disorder includes:

- Endometrial hyperplasia or cancer
- Endometriosis
- Polycystic ovarian syndrome
- Dysfunctional uterine bleeding (heavy or prolonged)

Gynecological disorders affect the internal and the external organs in the female pelvic and abdominal areas. These disorders include dysmenorrhea (pain associated with menstruation,) Vulvodynia (unexplained chronic discomfort or pain of the vulva,) and chronic pelvic pain (a persistent and severe pain occurring primarily in the lower abdomen.)

Some problems can affect the proper functioning of the reproductive system and may affect a woman's ability to get pregnant. One example, *polycystic ovary syndrome*, occurs when immature follicles in the ovaries form together to create a large cyst, ultimately preventing mature eggs from being released. Another reproductive disorder, *endometriosis*, occurs when the type of tissue that lines the uterus grows elsewhere, such as on the ovaries or other abdominal organs. Uterine fibroids are non-cancerous tumors that grow in the uterine cavity, within the wall of the uterus, or on the outside of the uterus.

ENDOMETRIAL HYPERPLASIA

Endometrial hyperplasia is a condition in which the *endometrium* (lining of the uterus) is abnormally thick.

There are four types of endometrial hyperplasia.

The types vary by the number of abdominal cells and the presence of cell changes. *These types are*:

- Simple endometrial hyperplasia
- Complex endometrial hyperplasia
- Simple atypical endometrial hyperplasia
- Complex atypical endometrial hyperplasia.

Symptoms of Endometrial Hyperplasia

The primary symptoms of endometrial hyperplasia is abdominal menstrual bleeding.

Contact your doctor if you experience the following:

- Menstrual bleeding that is heavier or longer lasting than usual.
- Menstrual bleeding between menstrual periods.
- Menstrual cycles (amount of time between periods) that are shorter than 21 days.
- Not having a period (pre-menopause).
- Post-menopause uterine bleeding.

Causes of Endometrial Hyperplasia

Endometrial hyperplasia is caused by too much estrogen or not enough progesterone. Both hormones play roles in the menstrual cycle. Estrogen makes the cells grow, while progesterone signals the shedding of the cells. A hormonal imbalance can produce too many cells or abnormal cells.

Endometrial Hyperplasia Treatment

Treatment options for endometrial hyperplasia depends on what type you have. The most common treatment is with Progestin. This can be taken in several forms, including pills, shots, vaginal creams, or through intra-uterine devices. Your doctor will help you decide which treatment option is best for you.

UTERINE POLYPS

Uterine polyps, also called endometrial polyps, are small, soft growth on the inside of a woman's uterus, called the endometrium. They can range in size from as small as a sesame seed, to as large as a golf ball. You may have just one polyp or many of them at once. Most uterine polyps aren't cancerous. Many women don't have symptoms, and some don't need any treatment. But doctors have several ways to find and remove them.

Causes of Uterine Polyps

It may be linked to changes in hormone levels of the woman's body. Each month, your estrogen levels rise and fall, causing the lining of your uterus to thicken and then shed during your periods. Polyps form when too much of that lining grows.

Things Likely to be the cause of having polyps.

- **Age:** they're common in your 40s or 50s that may be due to the change in estrogen levels that happens just before and during menopause.
- **Obesity** If you have a high risk of obesity, high blood pressure, breast cancer or drug tamoxifen.

Symptoms

You may not have any symptoms, especially if you have small polyps or only one.

Talk to your doctor if you notice:

- Irregular periods, when you can't predict their timing, length or heaviness.
- Heavy periods.
- Bleeding or spotting between periods.
- Vaginal bleeding after menopause.
- Trouble with getting pregnant.

Polyps can also cause problems with fertility. They may keep you from getting pregnant or make you more likely to miscarry. That's because they can keep a fertilized egg from attaching to your uterus or block your fallopian tubes or cervix. Some studies have found that removing polyps can help women get pregnant. But there isn't any clear proof that it works for everyone.

Treatment

Depending on your case, your doctor might recommend the following:

- **Watchful waiting**: You may not need treatment if you don't have any symptoms and the polyps isn't cancerous. It might go away on its own. But if you're past menopause or at a higher risk of uterine cancer, your doctor will remove it.
- **Medications**. Progestin and Gonadotrop in releasing hormone agonists, help control your hormone levels. They may shrink polyps and ease symptoms, like heavy bleeding. But the symptoms often return when you stop taking the drug.
- **Surgery**. Doctors can usually remove polyps during the same procedures they use to diagnose them, such as hysteroscopy or curettage. Instead of making a cut in your belly, they can insert a curette or other surgical tools through your vagina and cervix to take the polyps out. If your polyps have cancer cells, you may need surgery to take out your entire uterus in a process that's called hysterectomy.

UTERINE POLYPS VS FIBROIDS

Polyps and Fibroid are similar, but there are a few differences. Fibroids are overgrowths of the muscle inside the walls of your uterus, not the tissue lining inside. Like polyps, they can cause heavy bleeding. But they can also cause pain, constipation and trouble with urinating.

Prevention

There's no sure way to prevent uterine polyps. Losing extra weight might help lower the risks of having them. Polyps can come back, so get regular checkups from your doctor if you have had treatment.

ENDOMETRIOSIS

Endometriosis is a disorder in which tissue that normally lines the uterus grows outside the uterus. With endometriosis, the tissue can be found on the ovaries, the fallopian tubes or the intestines.

Symptoms include the following:

- Pain and menstrual irregularities. Pain (usually pelvic) that occurs just before menstruation which lessens after menstruation.
- Pain while having sexual intercourse.
- Cramping during sex.
- Cramping or pain during bowel movements or urination.
- Infertility.
- Pain with pelvic examinations.

Getting pregnant and having a healthy baby are possible and common with endometriosis. Having endometriosis may make it more difficult for you to conceive than women without this condition. It may also increase your risk for serious pregnancy complications. Pregnant women with the condition are considered high risk.

Endometriosis has no cure, but its symptoms can be managed. Medical and surgical options are available to help reduce your symptoms and manage any potential complications. Your doctor may first try conservative treatment. Then may recommend surgery if your condition doesn't improve.

Danazol is a medication used in stopping menstruation and the symptoms. While taking *Danazol*, the disease may continue to progress. Danazol can have side effects, including acne and hirsutism. Hirsutism is abnormal hair growth on your face and body.

POLYCYSTIC OVARY SYNDROME

This is a hormonal disorder causing enlarged ovaries with small cysts on the outer edges. It affects up to 27% of women of child-bearing age. The cause of polycystic ovary syndrome isn't well known, but it may involve a combination of genetic and environmental factors.

Symptoms include the following:

- Menstrual irregularity
- Excess hair growth
- Acne
- Obesity

Women with PCOS produce higher-than-normal amounts of male hormones. This hormone-imbalance causes them to skip menstrual periods and make it harder for them to get pregnant. It involves cysts in the ovaries.

PCOS may also cause hair growth on the face and body and may also provoke female baldness. It can contribute to long-term health problems like diabetes and heart disease. Women with PCOS often have increased levels of inflammation in their body.

Studies have linked excess inflammation to higher androgen levels. It also provokes dark patches of skin to form in body creases like those on the neck, in the groin and under the breast.

It is also linked to the following:

Heavy bleeding: The uterine lining builds up for a longer time, so the periods you do get can be heavier than normal.

Infertility: To get pregnant, you have to ovulate. Women who don't ovulate regularly don't release as many eggs to be fertilized. PCOS is one of the leading causes of infertility in women.

Weight loss and other treatments can improve your odds of having a healthy pregnancy.

Treatment for PCOS

It usually starts with life changes like weight loss, diet, and exercise. Studies comparing diets for PCOS have found that low carbohydrate diets are effective for both weight loss and lowering insulin levels. A low glycemic index; (low GI) diet that gets most carbohydrate from fruits, vegetables, and whole grains helps regulate the menstrual cycle.

Exercise

Studies have found that 30 minutes of moderate intensive exercise at least three days a week can help women with PCOS lose weight. Losing weight with exercise also improves ovulation and insulin levels.

Exercise is even more beneficial when combined with a healthy diet. Diet plus exercise helps you lose more weight, than either intervention alone, and it lowers the risk of diabetes and heart disease. All these combined with a balance of positive and negative polarity of the Vital Life Force goes a long way to help.

Birth control pills and the diabetes drug; Metformin, can help bring back a normal menstrual cycle. Cellophane and surgery improve fertility in women with PCOS. See your doctor if you have skipped periods or you have other PCOS symptoms, or you have been trying to get pregnant in the last 12 months or more without success.

INFERTILITY

Infertility is the inability to conceive within a 12 month period. We generally recommend seeking the help of a reproductive endocrinologist if conception has not occurred within 12 months of trying. However, there are times where one may be advised to seek help earlier.

These include:

Infrequent Menstrual Periods

When a woman has regular menstrual periods; defined as regular cycle, occurring every 21 to 35 days, this almost always indicates that she ovulates regularly. Ovulation of the egg occurs approximately 2 weeks before the start of the next period. If a woman has cycles at intervals of greater than 35 days, it may indicate that she is not ovulating an egg predictably, or even at all. Ovulation of the egg is essential for pregnancy.

Therefore, we recommend a re-evaluation of the menstrual cycle, if infrequent or irregular in a couple attempting pregnancy.

Females Aged 35 or Older

Egg numbers decrease at a rapid rate as a woman grows older. Furthermore, as aging occurs, egg quality, or the likelihood of an egg being genetically normal, decreases. Therefore, we recommend a fertility evaluation if a couple has been attempting pregnancy for 6 months or more when the woman is 35 years or older.

Sexually Transmitted Infection

Sexually transmitted infections such as chlamydia or gonorrhea, can cause inflammation and permanent scaring of the fallopian tubes. The opening of the fallopian tubes is essential for natural conception to take place, as the sperm must traverse the tubes in order to reach and fertilize the ovulated egg.

Uterine Fibroids or Endometrial Polyps

Uterine abnormalities, such as fibroids that indent the endometrial cavity and endometrial polyps, can impair how the endometrium (the lining of the uterus) and embryo interact to lower implementation and pregnancy rates. These abnormalities can also cause irregular bleeding between menstrual cycles. The main approach to correcting or removing these uterine abnormalities is by hysteroscopy; a surgical procedure whereby a narrow scope with a camera is placed within the uterine cavity.

Male Semen Abnormalities

If a male partner has a history of infertility with a prior partner, or if there are abnormalities on his semen analysis, then we advise earlier fertility evaluation. Ideally this should take place within 6 months of attempting pregnancy.

Endometriosis

Endometriosis is found in approximately 10 to 50% women of reproductive age and can be associated with infertility. As earlier described, it can also cause pain during intercourse and or menstrual periods.

TREATMENT FOR INFERTILITY

- **Education:** We strongly believe that educating women about the normal process of fertility, the problems that affect fertility, and the treatment options will empower them to make the best choices for their reproductive health. Understanding the normal reproductive process is essential in knowing when to seek help.
- **Medications to Induce Egg Development and Ovulation:** The medications that help stimulate the ovaries to develop mature eggs for ovulation come in two forms; pills taken orally (by mouth) or injections. The most commonly prescribed pill to stimulate ovulation is *Clomiphene Citrate.* This pill is

generally taken from menstrual cycle days, 3 - 7. The most prescribed injections that stimulate the ovaries are called *Gonadotropins*. These injections are taken nightly; typically for 5 - 10 days. They act directly on the cells of the ovaries, to stimulate egg development. Once a follicle containing an egg reaches a mature size, another hormone injection called the *Human Chorionic Gonadotropin* or HCG, is what is usually given, to mimic the natural LH surge (Luteinizing Hormone) that occurs at the time of ovulation. This leads to the final maturation and release of the egg.

- **Insemination**. Intra-uterine insemination; also known as IUI is a process by which sperm is washed and prepared for placement into the uterine cavity, therefore by passing the cervix and bringing a higher concentration of motile sperm closer to the tubes and ovulated egg.
- **In Vitro Fertilization (IVF)** In Vitro means "outside the body". Usually referred to as IVF, it is a process whereby eggs are collected and then fertilized by sperm outside the human body in an embryology laboratory.
- **Third party reproduction** This is a reference to a general process where another person provides sperm or egg, or where another woman acts as a gestational surrogate, with the purpose of helping another person or couple have a child.
- **Surgery** In reproductive medicine, the most common surgical procedures are Laparoscopy, hysteroscopy, and abdominal myomectomy (removal of Uterine fibroids).

Do You Want to Give Birth to an Active Brilliant Child?

Are you finding it difficult to conceive? If you said "yes" to either one, then the book, "*Let Nature Help You Nurture,*" is a miracle book for you. This book represents the definitively revolutionary, clinically proven, and natural system for conceiving fast. It explains how we may take advantage of the positive periods of the moon's tide to conceive a brilliant active child, and likewise, points out those periods that can produce weak children and slow learners.

This book gives you the key to understanding infertility disorders, restoring hormonal balances, and enhancing reproductive health by addressing the root cause of infertility. Thus, it will help you to conceive and give birth to a healthy brilliant and active baby faster than you ever thought possible. Regardless of your age, how long you have tried to conceive or how severe or chronic your infertility disorder is, there is hope for you.

All prospective parents should read the book, *"Let Nature Help You Nurture."*

Link: https://www.amazon.com/dp/B08134PB8T

About the Author

Charles Tita was born on the 12th of June 1957 in Bali, Bamenda, in the north-west region of Cameroon.

From his youth he thirsted to know the truth about the Mystery of our Universe. At an early age, he was eager to attend the Senior Seminary but his father, a senior politician and statesman serving in the country's parliament would never allow his first son to become a priest, because he had only two sons and fourteen daughters. Over his dead body would the old man allow his first son to become a priest. For Charles, even if the world came to an end, the young lad was determined to become a priest.

In 1978 when his father stubbornly refused to sign his novitiate form to allow Charles to continue in the Seminary, Charles left the Senior Seminary and joined the Saint Bernard's Monastery in Mbengwi. Here he found certain manuscripts which had been greatly guarded, concealed and hidden for millennia. Hidden knowledge that the public is searching for to live a happy and successful lives. Charles was determined to learn by heart, all this hidden knowledge which were discussed in private whispered tones and passed down only from a master to a close initiate in moments of extreme trust. After much reflection Charles decided to study by heart these hidden secret knowledge in other to be of service to others who were seeking what he had found. He knew there was great thirst and hunger by others to benefit from what he had found.

He later joined the Saint John of God hospital in Nguti where he could use this knowledge to help the sick.

The following year Charles started writing. His first manuscript was like Charles writing his own death warrant. Before this time, no person had ever dare to reveal this guarded knowledge.

Charles was summoned by the council of Abbott to recant his writings, and to hand over the manuscript to be burnt. When Charles had refused to hand over the manuscript, he was declared a non-grata.

At midnight, Charles was kidnapped and ferried to Nigeria. This was during the outbreak of the Severe Acute Respiratory syndrome (SARs COV-Z), an epidemy linked to the highly infection corona virus, in the 2000s.

It was thought that Charles would die here. But instead, he became a key player in eradicating the virus.

In 2012 during the outbreak of the 2012 Middle East Respiratory syndrome (MERS), Charles won an award for the several manuscripts he wrote on how to prevent, contain and eradicate the disease.

Though Charles prefers to remain unknown, this philosopher, scientist, educator and author stands out as one of the beacons among the world's most illustrious torch-bearers of the twenty-first century.

www.ingramcontent.com/pod-product-compliance
Ingram Content Group UK Ltd.
Pitfield, Milton Keynes, MK11 3LW, UK
UKHW041844200726
13854UKWH00005BA/2064

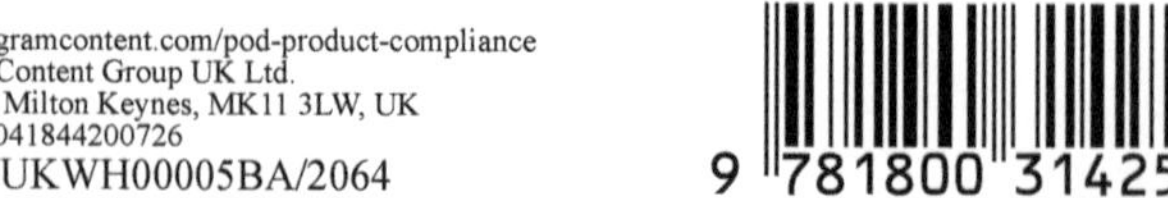